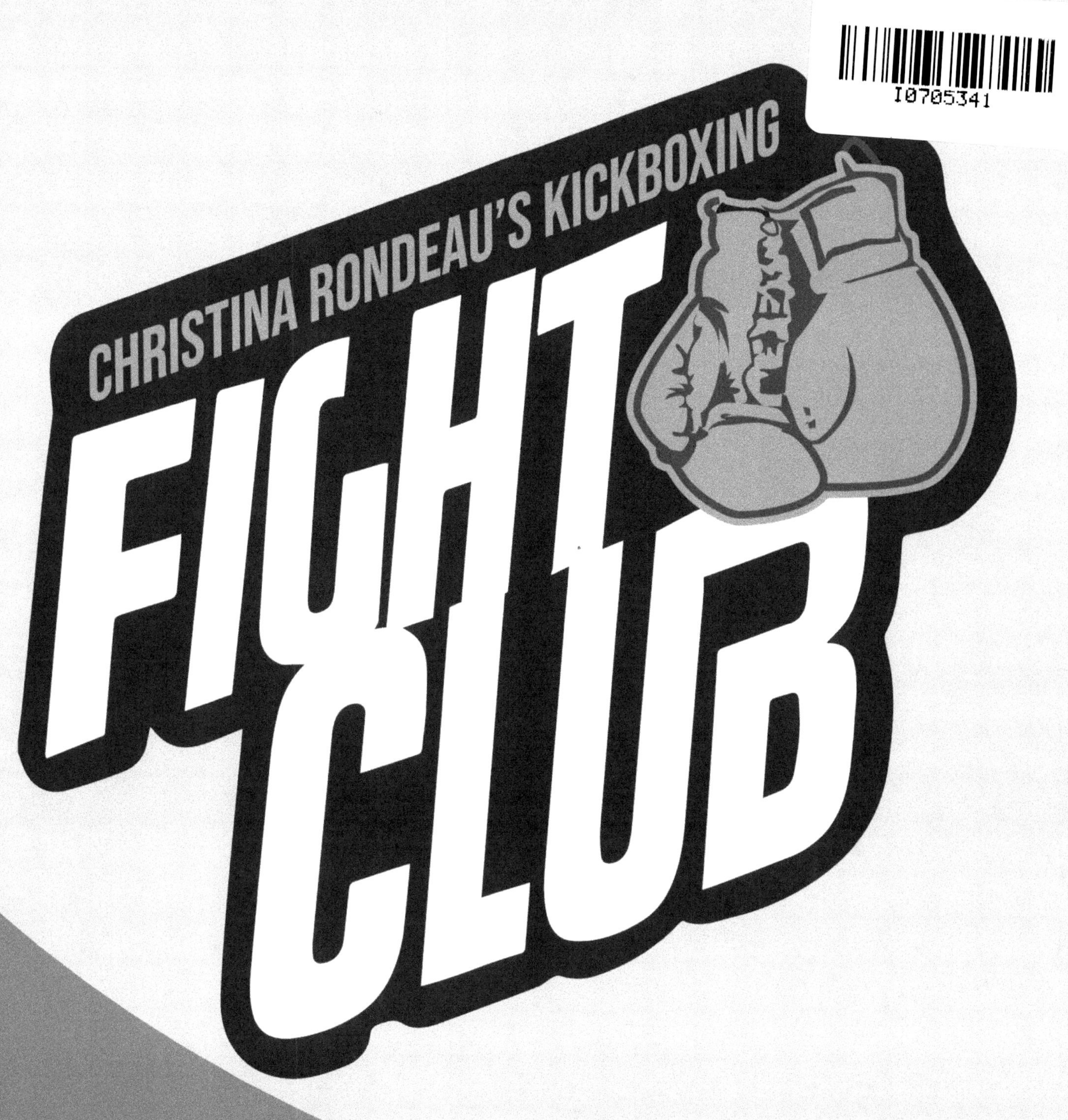

10 Round Circuit Training

Workouts and Drills

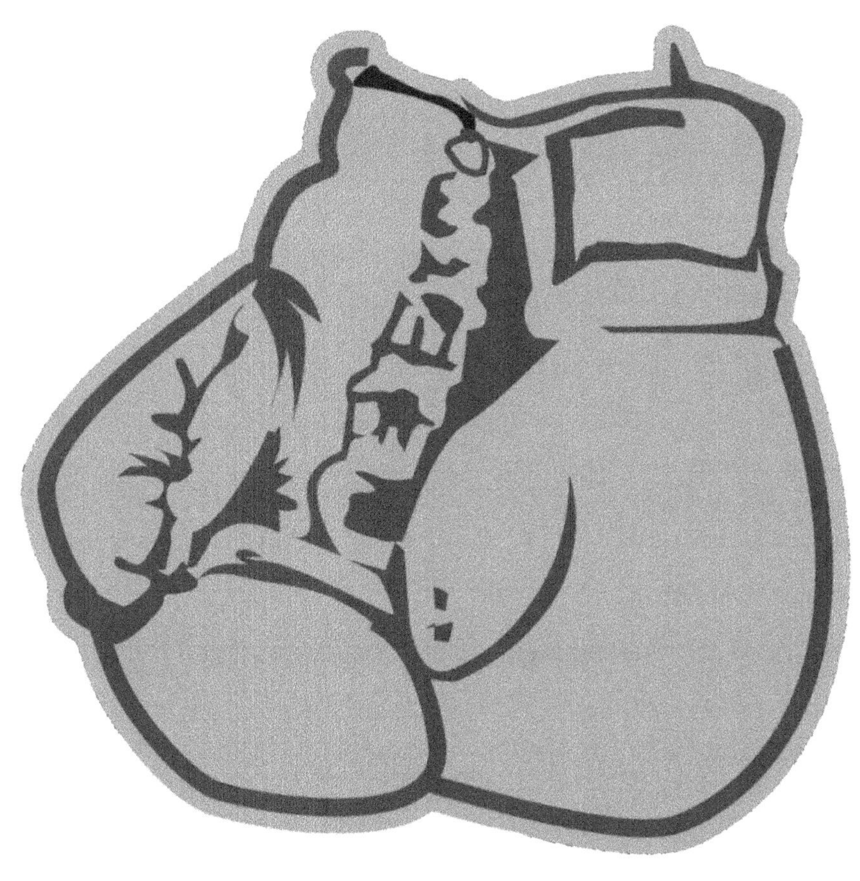

This book belongs to

____

TEAM - FAMILY

Christina Rondeau's Kickboxing Corporation is a family, community, friendship and a team.

We honor the fighter in everyone, not just physically but what people fight through on this life journey. Mind, Body, and Soul is developed through physical, mental, and emotional training. Creator and Founder, Christina Rondeau, has created *Fight Club 10 Round Circuit Training* to allow others to be a part of this team and own their own facility through our licensing program. This model revolutionizes being an owner through freedom. Owners will have the freedom they want and need but still be a part of the brand with the professional expertise to back it and especially be part of this amazing team! We want to help others' mind, body, and soul grow, and by having Fight Clubs all over the world, we can do that! Contact our team today to find out how you can own a "Fight Club" at info@rkblive.com

www.ChristinaRondeau.com
401-996-5425

COMMUNITY - FRIENDSHIP

This book was developed to help guide trainers with workouts. A big thank you to the trainers of Christina Rondeau Kickboxing Corporation for helping create these workouts for this book.

Bernadette Marshall, Danielle Scott, Hope Barrette, Rebecca Rhodes, Brittany Valentine, Laina Borowski and Laura Petrone

Thank you for being amazing trainers and part of everything CRKB stands for!

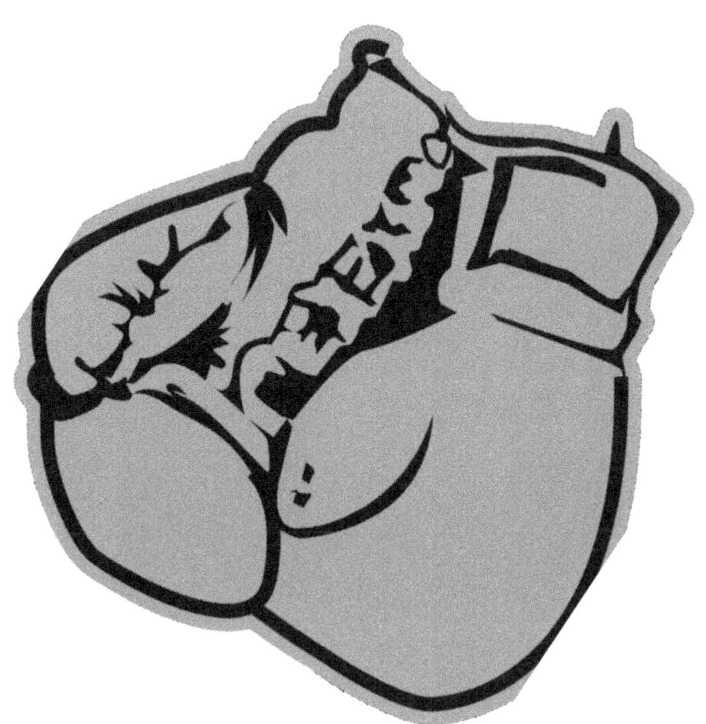

WORKOUT 1

Round 1 – Cardio
      20 Jumping Jacks
      10 Jump Squats

Round 2 – Weights (Shoulders & Biceps)
      15 Upright Rows
      15 Straight Bar Curls

Round 3 – Heavy Bag Round
      1,1, 2, 1, 2
      Shuffle
      6 Front Ball Kicks

Round 4 -Weights (Back & Bicep)
      12 Lat Pulldowns
      12 Bicep Curls

Round 5 – Heavy Bag
      1,2,3, 2
      Shuffle
      4 Front Punches (1,2,1,2)

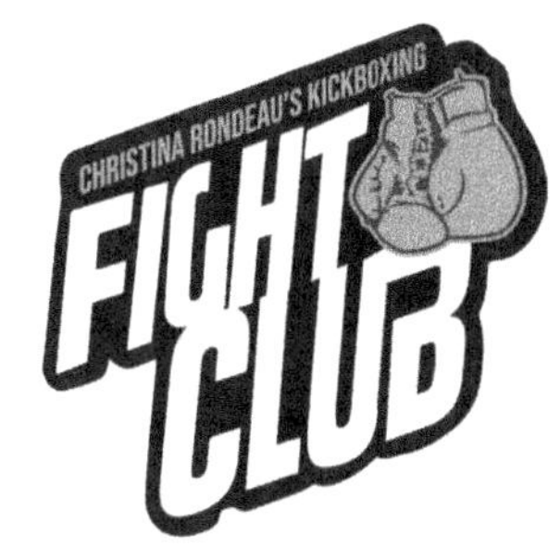

Round 6 - Speed Bag (Left Fighting Stance)
       5 L -5R
       3 L -3R
       1 L -1R

Round 7 – Heavy Bag Round
       1,2,3,6,3,2
       Shuffle
       4 Instep

Round 8 – Weights / Legs
       15 Alternating Leg Lunges
       15 Ice Skaters

Round 9 – Heavy Bag Round
       1,3,1,2,6,2
       Shuffle
       Double Jab

Round 10 – Abs
       20 Leg Lifts
       20 Bicycles

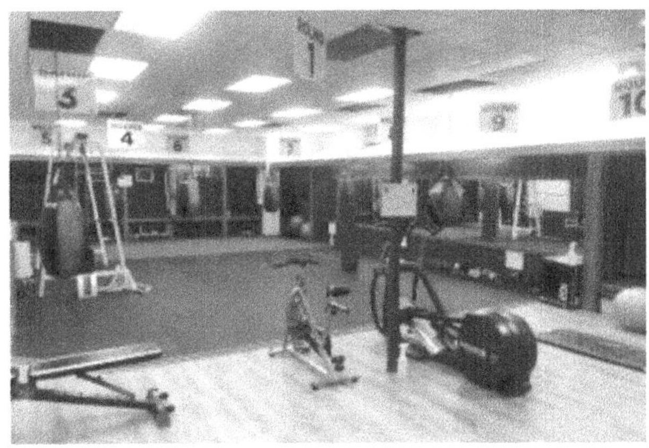

WORKOUT 2

Round 1 – Cardio
       Elliptical– Crank it out!

Round 2 – Weights (Chest and Triceps)
       15 Chest Press
       15 Overhead Tricep Extensions

Round 3 - Heavy Bag Round
       1,2,1,2
       Shuffle
       4 Instep Kicks

Round 4 - Weights (Back & Bicep)
       15 Rows
       15 Hammer Curls

Round 5 – Heavy Bag Rounds
       1,2,3,2
       Shuffle
       4 Front Ball Kicks (Alternating Legs)

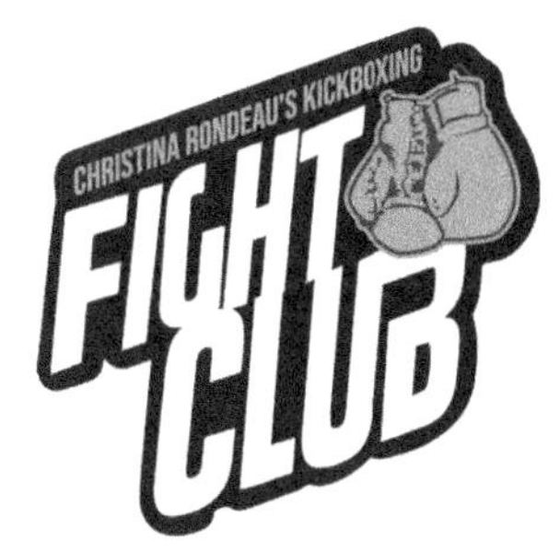

Round 6 - Speed Bag (Left Fighting Stance)
        Left Hand 10
        Right Hand 10

Round 7 – Heavy Bag Round
        1,2,3,6,3,2
        Shuffle
        LRH, RRH, LRH

Round 8 – Weights (With Band)
        10 Hip Abductor
        10 Glute Extensions
        10 Alternating Side Lunges

Round 9 –Heavy Bag Round
        20 Straight Punches
        Shuffle
        LRH, L Side Kick, R Front Ball Kick

Round 10 – Abs
        25 Crunches
        25 Leg Lifts
        25 Russian Twists

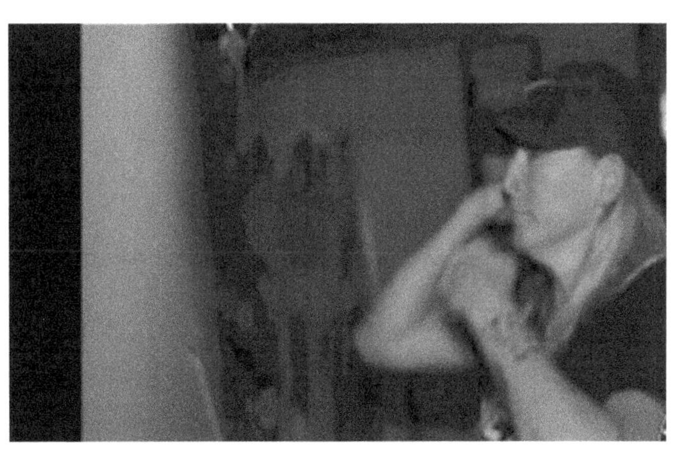

WORKOUT 3

Round 1 – Cardio
      20 Ice Skates
      20 Squats
      20 Jumping Jacks

Round 2 – Weights (Chest & Triceps)
      15 Chest Press
      15 Skull Crushers

Round 3 – Heavy Bag Round
      1,1,1 (Triple Jab)
      Shuffle
      6 Instep Kicks

Round 4-Weights (Back & Bicep)
      12 Upright Rows
      12 Hammer Curls

Round 5 – Heavy Bag
      10 Punches
      Shuffle
      4 Alternating Instep Kicks

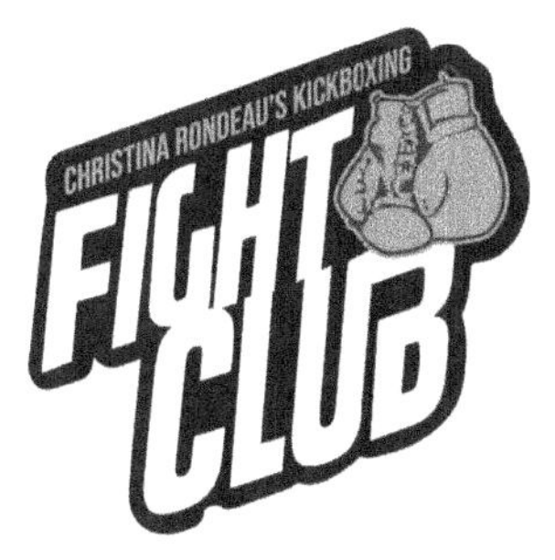

Round 6 - Speed Bag (Left Fighting Stance)
      Left Hand 10
      Right Hand 10

Round 7 – Heavy Bag Round
      1,1,2,1,2
      Shuffle
      3 Left RH

Round 8 – Weights
      20 Ball Slams
      20 Toe Taps

Round 9 – Heavy Bag Round
      1, 2, 3, 2, 1, 2, 3, 2
      Shuffle
      Double Jab

Round 10 – Abs
      10 Full Sit ups
      20 Crunches
      20 Heel Reaches

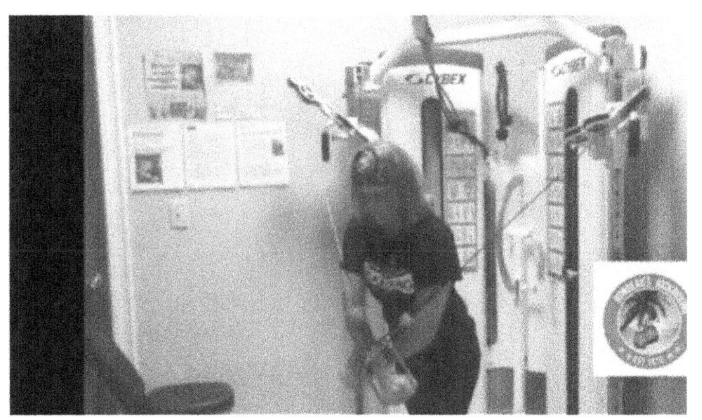

WORKOUT 4

Round 1 – Cardio
       25 Bicycles
       20 Butt Kicks
       10 Burpees

Round 2 – Weights (Chest & Tricep)
       15 Chest Flies
       15 Tricep Kick Backs

Round 3 – Heavy Bag Round
       10 Straight Punches
       Shuffle
       4 Instep

Round 4 -Weights (Shoulder & Biceps)
       15 Lateral Raise
       15 Hammer Curls

Round 5 – Heavy Bag
       1,3,1 2,4,2
       Shuffle
       10 Instep

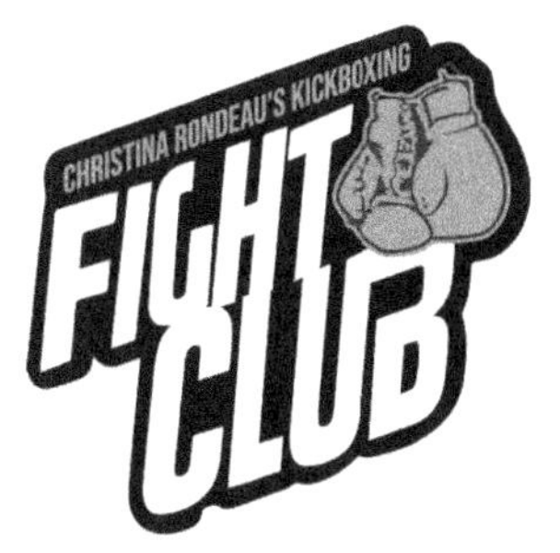

Round 6 - Speed Bag (Left Fighting Stance)
>   3 Left
>   3 Right

Round 7 – Heavy Bag Round
>   1, 1, 2, 3, 2
>   Shuffle
>   4 Punches

Round 8 – Weights
>   15 Squat Curl Press w/weights
>   15 Alternating Leg Lunges w/weights

Round 9 – Heavy Bag Round
>   1, 2, 3, LRH, 2
>   Shuffle
>   LRH, R Front Ball Kick, LRH

Round 10 – Abs
>   20 Butterfly Crunches
>   20 Dead Bugs
>   20 Heel Taps

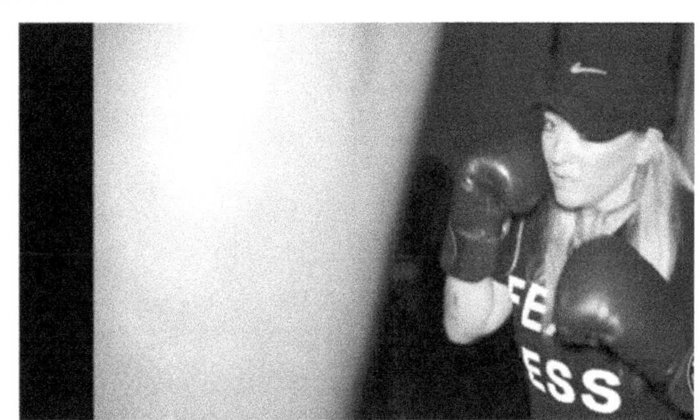

WORKOUT 5

Round 1 – Cardio
       20 Jumping Jacks
       10 Jump Squats
       20 Jumping Lunges

Round 2 – Weights (Back & Bicep)
       15 Bent Over Rows
       15 Bicep Curls

Round 3 – Heavy Bag Round
       1, 2, 3, 4, 3, 2
       Shuffle
       4 Instep Kicks

Round 4 -Weights (Back & Shoulders)
       10 Lat Pull Downs
       20 Rope Slams

Round 5 – Heavy Bag
       LRH, LRH, 2,3,2
       Shuffle
       1,2,1,2

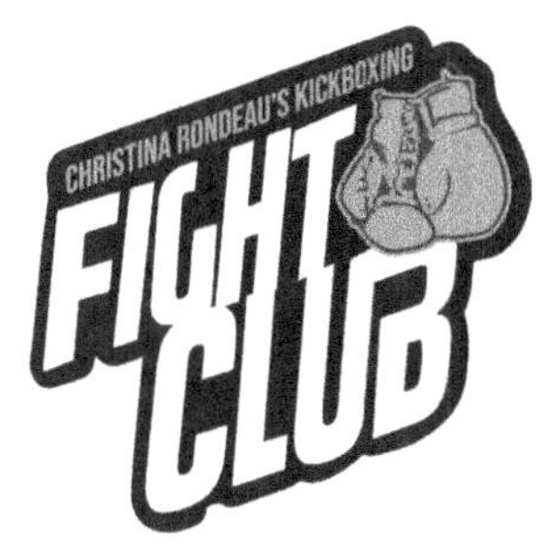

Round 6 - Speed Bag (Left Fighting Stance)
        5 Left
        5 Right

Round 7 – Heavy Bag Round
        1, 2, R-Side Hammer, L Side Hammer, 2,3,2
        Shuffle
        Double Jab

Round 8 – Weights
        15 Ball Smashes
        30 Toe Taps

Round 9 - Heavy Bag Round
        1, 2, 3, 6, 3, 2
        Shuffle
        RRH, RRH, RRH

Round 10 – Abs
        25 Butterfly Crunches
        10 Heel Taps

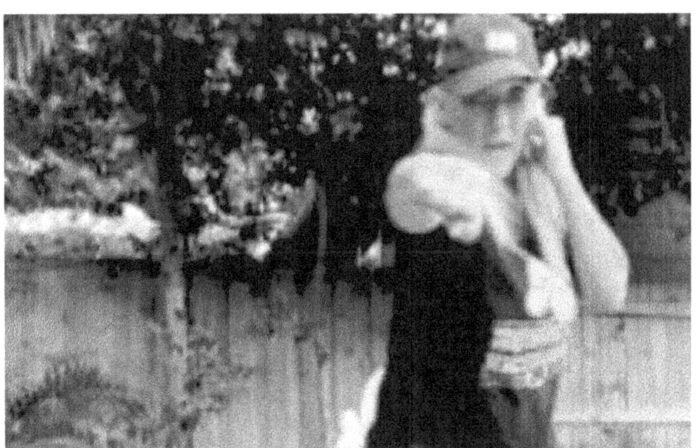

WORKOUT 6

Round 1 – Cardio
    20 Jumping Jacks
    10 Alternating Lunges
    15 Squats

Round 2 – Weights (Chest and Triceps)
    15 Chest Press
    15 Overhead Tricep Extension

Round 3 – Heavy Bag Round
    1, 2, 3, 2, Right Elbow
    Shuffle
    10 Punches

Round 4 -Weights (Back & Biceps)
    15 Lat Pull Downs
    15 Straight Bar Curl

Round 5 – Heavy Bag
    1, 5, LRH 2
    Shuffle
    4 Front Ball Kicks

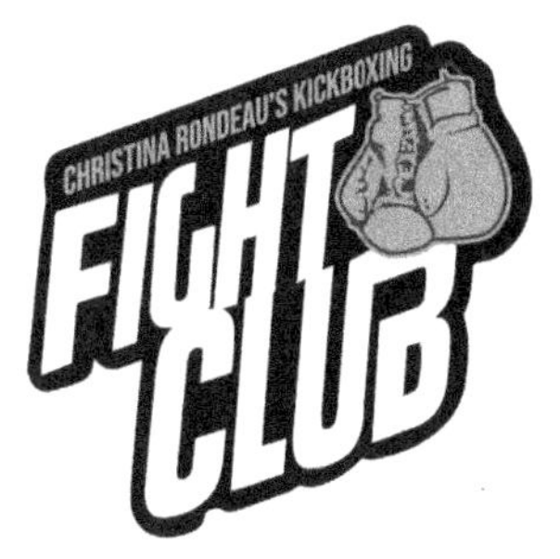

Round 6 - Speed Bag (Left Fighting Stance)
>10 Left Hand
>10 Right Hand

Round 7 – Heavy Bag Round
>1, 3, 1, 2, 4, 2
>Shuffle
>20 Punches

Round 8 – Weights - Shoulders
>15 Kettlebell Swings
>15 One arm Kettlebell Military Press (each arm)

Round 9 – Heavy Bag Round
>1, 2, 3, 2, 3, 2
>Shuffle
>LRH, R Ball Kick, LRH

Round 10 – Abs
>15 Sit ups
>15 Leg Lifts
>Last 30 sec. plank

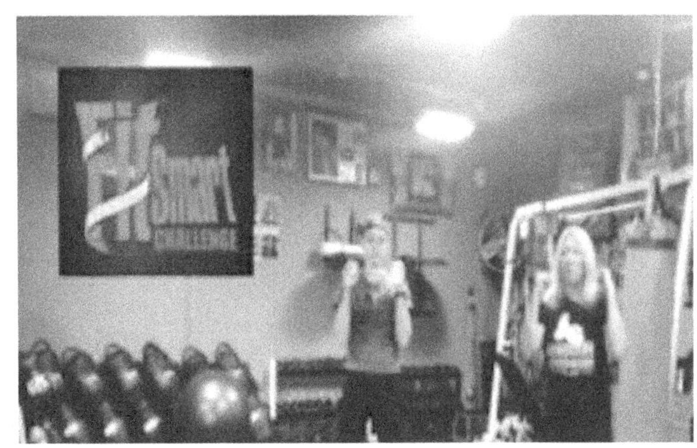

WORKOUT 7

Round 1 – Cardio
       20 Squats
       Alternate 20 Front Kicks

Round 2 – Weights (Back and Biceps)
       15 Single Arm Bent Rows
       15 Concentrated Bicep Curl

Round 3 – Heavy Bag Round
       1, 2, 3, 2, LRH LRH
       Shuffle
       Double Jab

Round 4 -Weights (Chest & Triceps)
       15 Cable Crossover
       15 Tricep Cable Press Down (1 arm)

Round 5 – Heavy Bag
       1,1,2,3,2 RRH, RRH,
       Shuffle
       1, 2, 1, 2

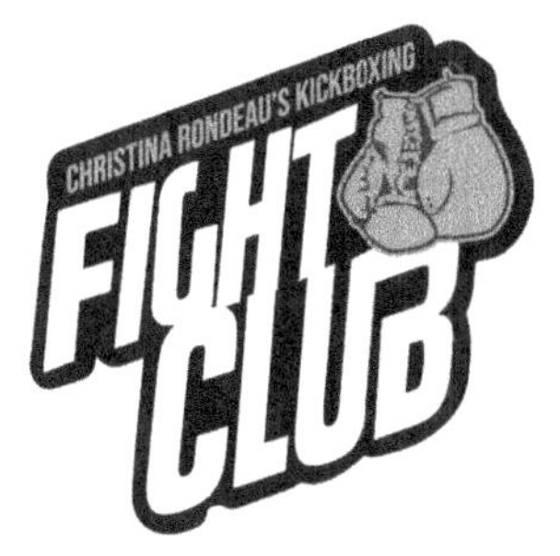

Round 6 - Speed Bag (Left Fighting Stance)
       5 Left
       5 Right

Round 7 – Heavy Bag Round
       1, 2, 3, 4,3,2
       Shuffle
       4 Instep Kicks

Round 8 – Weights
       20 Ball Smashes
       20 Quick Feet Ball Taps

Round 9 – Heavy Bag Round
       LRH, L-Side Kick, LRH, LRH
       Shuffle
       1, 2, 3, 6, 3,2

Round 10 – Abs
       20 Bicycles
       20 Crunches

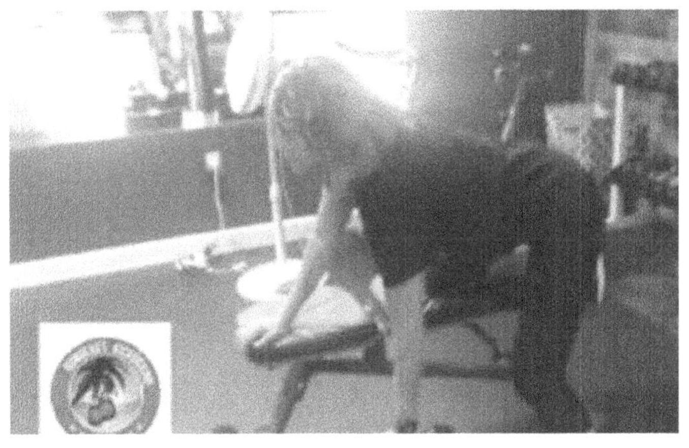

WORKOUT 8

Round 1 – Cardio
       Elliptical

Round 2 – Weights (Chest)
       12 Chest Press
       12 Chest Fly's

Round 3 – Heavy Bag Round
       1, 1, 2, 1, 2
       Shuffle
       6 Instep Kicks

Round 4 -Weights (Back & Bicep)
       12 Face Pulls
       12 Bicep Curls

Round 5 – Heavy Bag
       1,2, 3, 2, 2
       Shuffle
       LRH x3

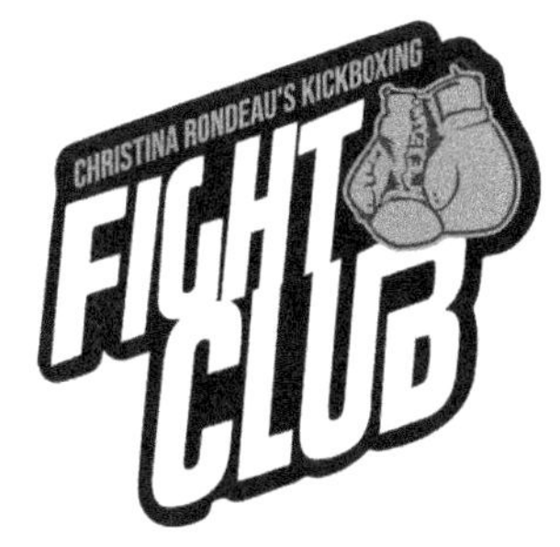

Round 6 - Speed Bag (Left Fighting Stance)
    20 Right
    20 Left

Round 7 – Heavy Bag Round
    1, 3, 1, 2, 6, 2
    Shuffle
    20 Punches

Round 8 – Weights
    15 Squat Curl Press
    15 Bicep Curls

Round 9 – Heavy Bag Round
    1, 2, 3, 6, 3, 2
    Shuffle
    4 Front Ball Kicks

Round 10 – Abs
    Slow Bicycles
    Hold Low Leg
      Lift last 30 sec.

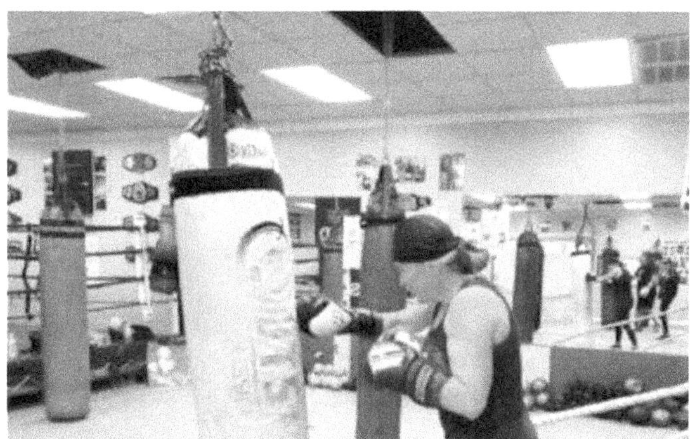

WORKOUT 9

Round 1 – Cardio
- 10 Jumping Jacks
- 10 Front Kicks Alternating

Round 2 – Weights (Shoulders)
- 15 Front Lateral Raises
- 15 Shoulder Shrugs

Round 3 – Heavy Bag Round
- 1, 2, 1, 2, 3, 2
- Shuffle
- LRH, RRH, LRH, 2

Round 4 -Weights (Arms)
- 15 Battle Rope Slams
- 15 Cable Upright Rows

Round 5 – Heavy Bag
- 1, 2, 1, 2   4, 4, 4, 4
- Shuffle
- 4 Front Ball Kicks

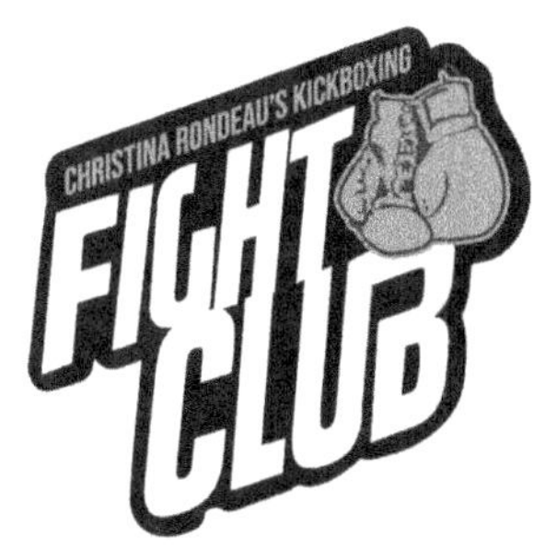

Round 6 - Speed Bag (Left Fighting Stance)
      20 Left
      20 Right
      20 Alternating

Round 7 – Heavy Bag Round
      LRH, 2,3, 3, 2   Shuffle
      3, 3, 6, 6

Round 8 – Heavy Bag Round
      1, 2, 1, 2, RRH, R Elbow
      Shuffle
      10 Punches

Round 9 – Weights
      15 Sumo Squats w/ Weights
      15 Alternating Leg Lunges with Bicep Curl

Round 10 – Abs
      10 Plank Shoulder Taps
      20 Russian Twists
      20 Crunches

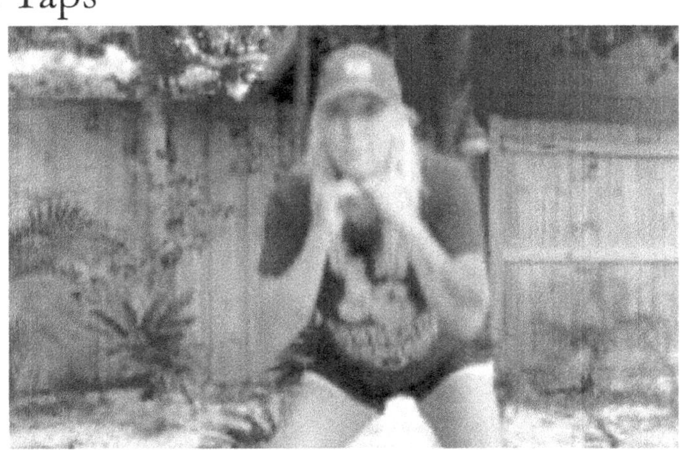

WORKOUT 10

Round 1 – Cardio
       20 Squats
       20 Alternating Lunges
       20 Curtsy Squats

Round 2 – Weights (Shoulders & Bicep)
       15 Military Press
       15 Bicep Curls

Round 3 – Heavy Bag Round
       1, 3, 1, 2, 6, 2
       Shuffle
       4 Instep

Round 4 -Weights (Back & Biceps)
       15Bar Lateral Pull Down
       15 Straight Bar Curl

Round 5 – Heavy Bag
       1, 2, 3, L Back Fist, 2
       Shuffle
       LRH, RRH, RRH, R Instep

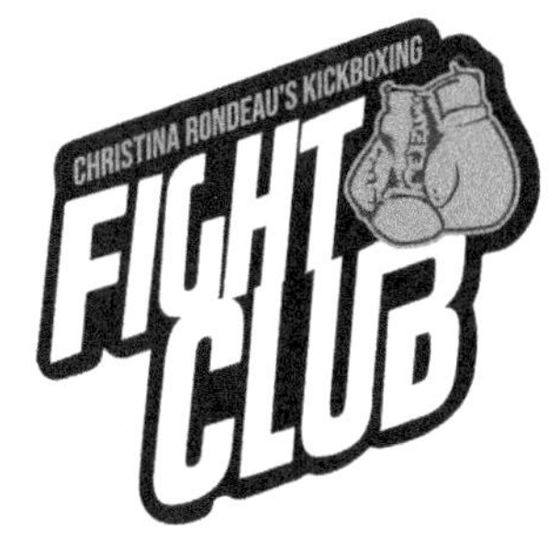

Round 6 - Speed Bag (Left Fighting Stance)
      3 L
      3 R

Round 7 – Heavy Bag Round
      LRH, LRH 2, 3, 3, 2
      Shuffle
      1, 2, 1, 2 Side Hammers x 4

Round 8 – Heavy Bag Round
      1, 2, 3, 2,3, 2
      Shuffle
      4 Straight Punches

Round 9 – Weights
      10 Squat Toss
      10 Ball Slams
      20 Toe Taps

Round 10 – Abs
      10 Crunches
        on ball
      20 Russian Twists
        w/ Ball

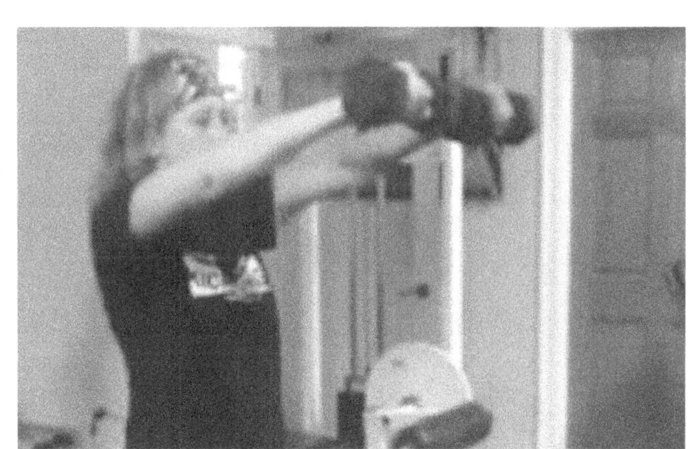

WORKOUT 11

Round 1 – Cardio
       Shadow Box- 3 Minutes

Round 2 – Weights (Back & Bicep)
       15 Back Row
       15 Bicep Curls

Round 3 – Heavy Bag Round
       1,1,2,3,2
       Shuffle
       6 Alternating Instep Kicks

Round 4 -Weights (Chest & Tricep)
       15 Push ups
       15 Tricep Push downs w/rope

Round 5 – Heavy Bag
       LRH, LRH, LRH 2, 3, 2, 3,2
       Shuffle
       10 Punches

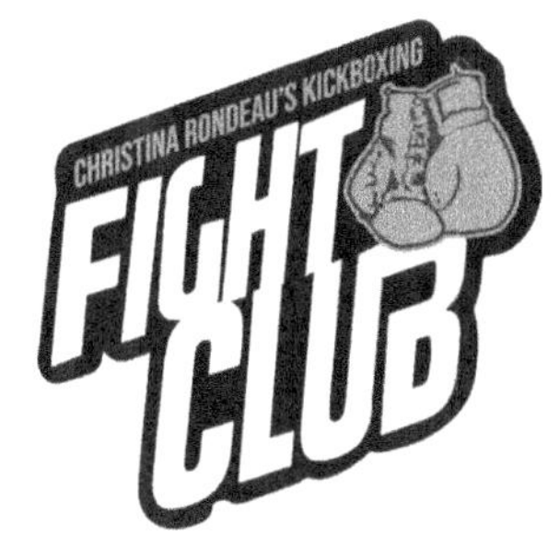

Round 6 - Speed Bag (Left Fighting Stance)
      10 L
      10 R

Round 7 – Heavy Bag Round
      1, 2, 3, 4, 3, 2
      LRH, LRH, LRH
      Shuffle
      2, 3, 2, 3,2

Round 8 – Heavy Bag Round
      LRH, R Front Ball Kick, RRH,
      Shuffle
      6,6,3,2

Round 9 – Weights
      20 Ball Slams
      20 Toe Taps

Round 10 – Abs
      20 Crunches
      20 Leg Raises
      20 Bicycles
      Plank for least
        30 sec.

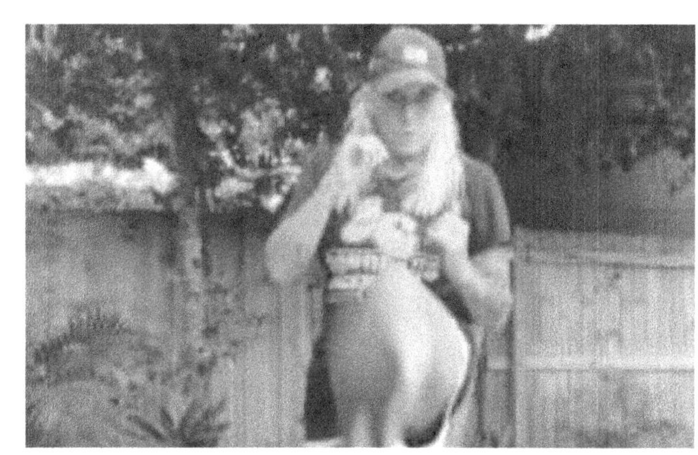

WORKOUT 12

Round 1 – Cardio
      30 Jumping Jacks
      30 Squats

Round 2 – Weights (Chest)
      15 Chest Press
      15 Chest Fly's

Round 3 – Heavy Bag Round
      1, 2, 3, 4, 3, 2
      Shuffle
      4 Front Ball Kicks

Round 4 -Weights (Triceps)
      15 Tricep Pull Downs
      15 Alternating Tricep Kickbacks

Round 5 – Heavy Bag
      1, 2, 1, 2, 4, 4, 4, 4
      Shuffle
      Double Jab

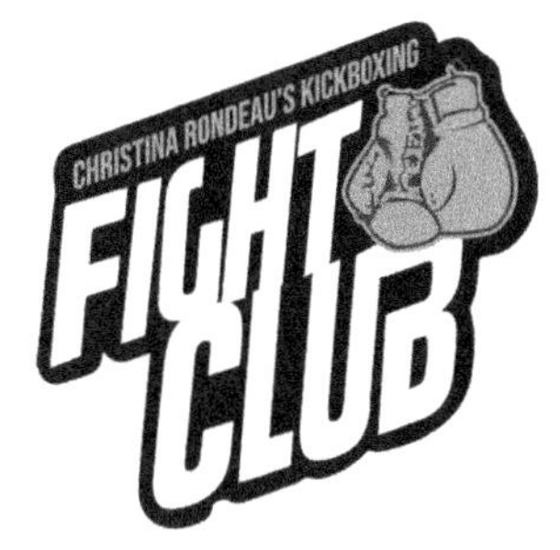

Round 6 - Speed Bag (Left Fighting Stance)
     3 L
     3 R

Round 7 – Heavy Bag Round
     1, 2, 3, 6, 3, 2
     Shuffle
     6 Alternating RH Kicks

Round 8 – Heavy Bag Round
     LRH, R Front Ball Kick, LRH 2,3,2
     Shuffle
     1, 2, 1, 2

Round 9 – Weights
     15 Squat Curl Press
     15 Alternating Leg Lunges Bicep Curl

Round 10 – Abs
     20 Cruches
     20 Leg Lifts
     Last 30 Seconds
        Knee to
        Elbow Plank

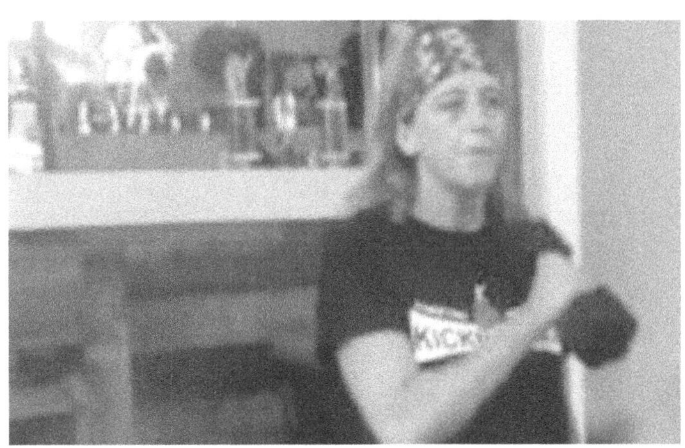

WORKOUT 13

Round 1 – Cardio
        20 High Knees
        20 Butt Kicks

Round 2 – Weights (Shoulders and Biceps)
        15 Upright Row
        15 Bicep Curls

Round 3 – Heavy Bag Round
        LRH LRH 2, 3, 2
        Shuffle
        6 Instep Kicks

Round 4 -Weights (Back and Biceps)
        15 Lat Pull Downs
        15 Straight Bar Curl

Round 5 – Heavy Bag
        1, 2, 3, 6, 3, 2
        Shuffle
        LRH, RRH, RRH, LRH

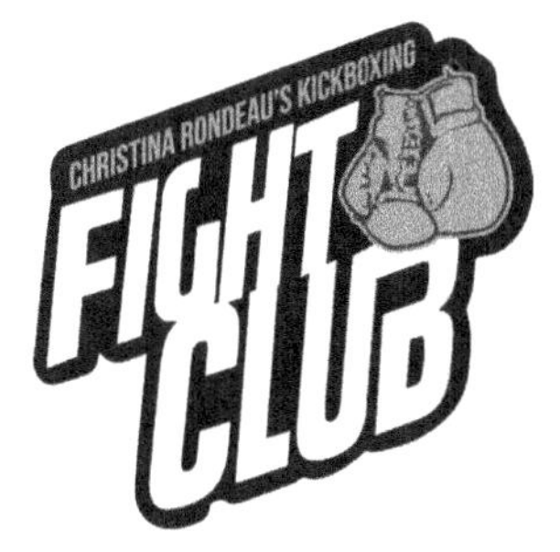

Round 6 - Speed Bag (Left Fighting Stance)
        20 R
        20 L

Round 7 – Heavy Bag Round
        1-2-3-5 LRH 2
        Shuffle
        10 Instep Kicks

Round 8 – Heavy Bag Round
        1, 2, 3, 2, 2, 2, R-Elbow
        Shuffle
        LRH, R Ball Kick, LRH

Round 9 – Weights
        15 Kettle Bell Raises
        15 1 Arm Kettle Bell Press

Round 10 – Abs
        20 Crunches
        20 Leg Lifts

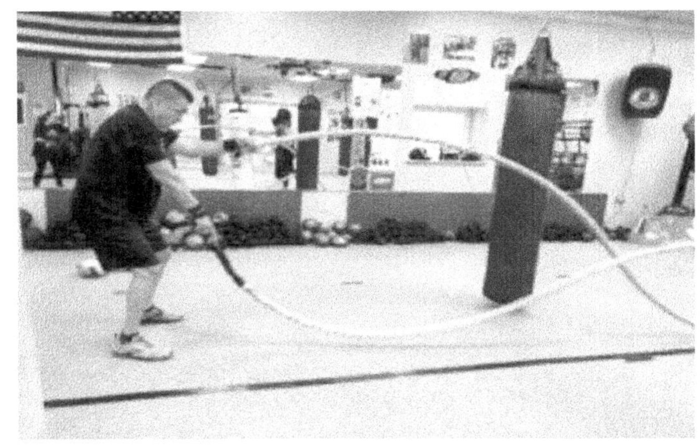

WORKOUT 14

Round 1 – Cardio
        20 Toe Taps
        10 Squats
        20 Butt Kickers

Round 2 – Weights (Chest & Tricep)
        12 Chest Press
        12 Tricep Kickbacks

Round 3 – Heavy Bag Round
        1, 3, 1, 4, 3, 2
        Shuffle
        1, 2, 1, 2

Round 4 -Weights (Back & Bicep)
        12 Back Fly's
        12 Bicep curls

Round 5 – Heavy Bag
        1, 5, LR 2
        Shuffle
        10 Punches

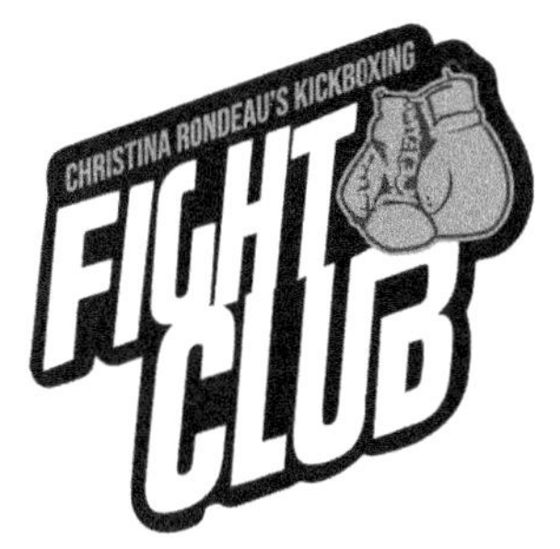

Round 6 - Speed Bag (Left Fighting Stance)
     5 L
     5 R
     3 L
     3 R

Round 7 – Heavy Bag Round
     1, slip to Right 2, 3, 2
     Shuffle
     LRH, RRH, LRH

Round 8 – Heavy Bag Round
     1, 2, 3 U, 3, 2
     Shuffle
     4 Front Ball Kicks

Round 9 – Weights
     20 Ice Skaters
     15 Dead Lifts

Round 10 – Abs
     20 Crunches
     20 Bicycles

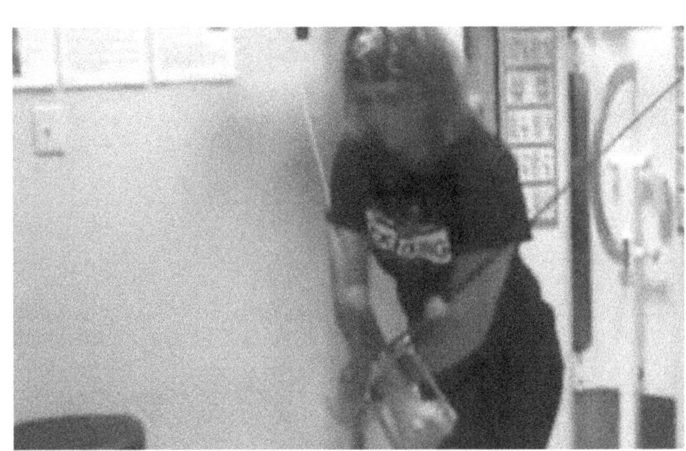

WORKOUT 15

Round 1 – Cardio
       20 High Knees
       20 Alternating High Kicks

Round 2 – Weights (Chest & Tri's)
       15 Chest Press
       15 Bench Dips

Round 3 – Heavy Bag Round
       1, 2, 3, 3, 2
       Shuffle
       LRH, RRH, LRH

Round 4 -Weights (Legs)
       Cable Pull Throughs
       Cable Romain Dead Lift

Round 5 – Heavy Bag
       1, 2, 3, 6, 3, 2
       Shuffle
       4 Stepping Stool Kicks

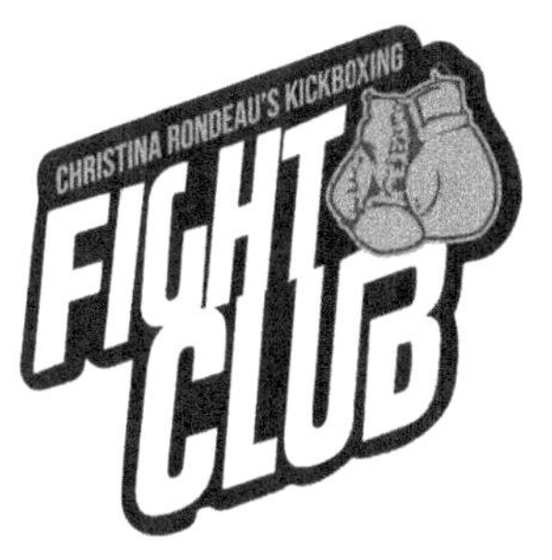

Round 6 - Speed Bag (Left Fight Stance)
       10 L
       10 R
       5 L
       5 R

Round 7 – Heavy Bag Round
       1, 2, 3, R Elbow x2
       Shuffle
       6 Instep Kicks

Round 8 – Heavy Bag Round
       5 Right Round House Kicks
       Switch Stance
       5 Left Round House Kicks

Round 9 – Weights – MMA BAG
       Flip 10 Times
       Toe Tops -50
       Ground and Pound! (Mix it up punches, elbows)

Round 10 – Abs
       50 Bicycles
       25 Crunches
       25 Leg Lifts

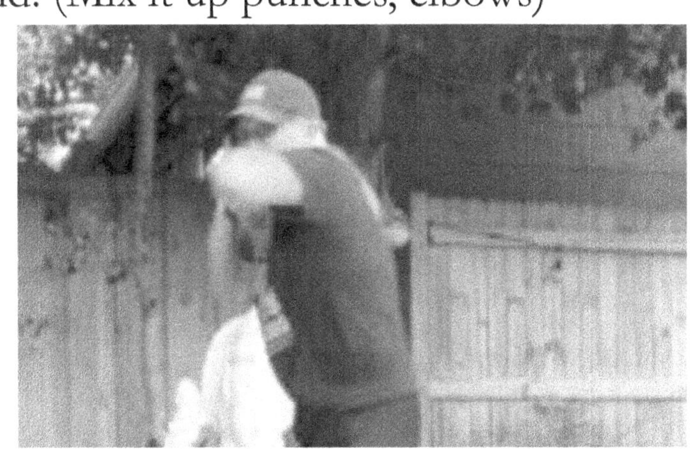

WORKOUT 16

Round 1 – Cardio
  Jump Rope / Ellipitical

Round 2 – Weights (Legs)
  15 Reverse Lunges w/ Weights
  15 Sumo Squats with Weight

Round 3 – Heavy Bag Round
  LRH, LRH, 2, 3, 4, 3, 2
  Shuffle
  4 Straight Punches

Round 4 -Weights (Back & Bicep)
  15 Lat Pull Down
  15 Straight Bar Curl

Round 5 – Heavy Bag
  LRH, L Instep Kick, LRH 2,3, 2
  Shuffle
  1, 2, 1, 2

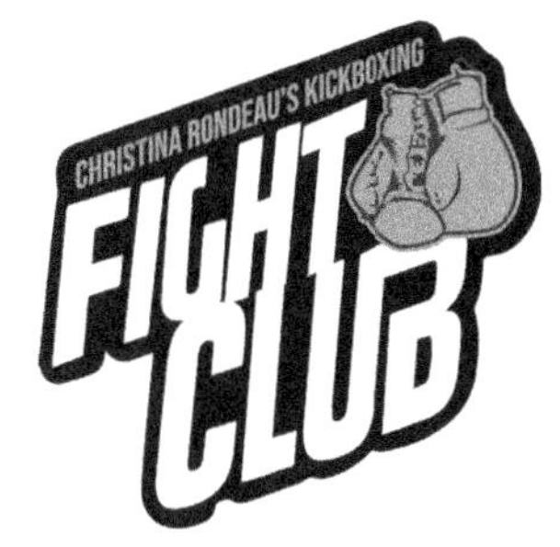

Round 6 - Speed Bag (Left Fighting Stance)
>Right Hand
>Down, Back, Punch

Round 7 – Heavy Bag Round
>1, 2, 3, 6, 3, 2
>Shuffle
>Right Round House Elbow – Left Forearm Elbow

Round 8 – Heavy Bag Round
>10 Cross Behind Side Kicks
>Shuffle
>20 Straight Punches

Round 9 – Weights (Shoulders & Bicep)
>15 Military Press
>15 Circular Bicep Curls

Round 10 – Abs
>20 Full Sit ups
>20 Leg Lifts
>20 Side Heel Taps
>last 30 sec. hold
>>leg lift 6 inches
>>off ground

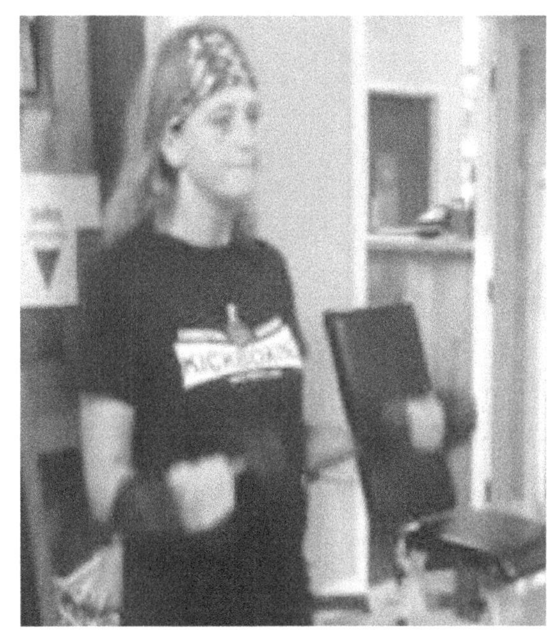

WORKOUT 17

Round 1 – Cardio
        30 Jumping Jacks
        30 Quick Feet Drop to a push up

Round 2 – Weights (Chest & Triceps)
        15 Overhead Chest Extensions
        10 Skull Crushers

Round 3 – Heavy Bag Round
        10 Straight Punches
        10 Instep Kicks

Round 4 -Weights (Back & Shoulder & Biceps)
        20 Trx Row with Squat
        20 Rope Slams

Round 5 – Heavy Bag
        1, 2, 3, 4, 4, 4, 4 (Alternating)
        Shuffle
        RRH, LRH, RRH

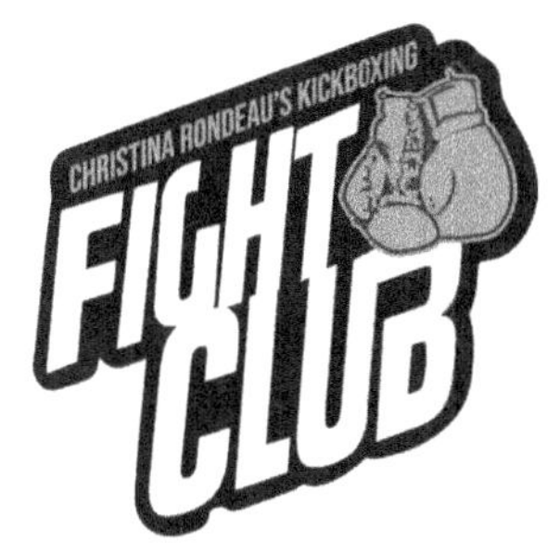

Round 6 - Speed Bag (Left Fighting Stance)
15 L
15 R
30 Alternating

Round 7 – Heavy Bag Round
1, 2, 3, 3, 6, 6, 3, 2
Shuffle
LRH, LRH, RRH, RRH

Round 8 – Heavy Bag Round
LRH, L-Sidekick, LRH 2,3,2
Shuffle
20 Punches

Round 9 – Weights
Ball Chest Press
Combo Shoulder Press Triceps Extension

Round 10 – Abs
20 Leg Lifts
20 Situps with
Russian Twists

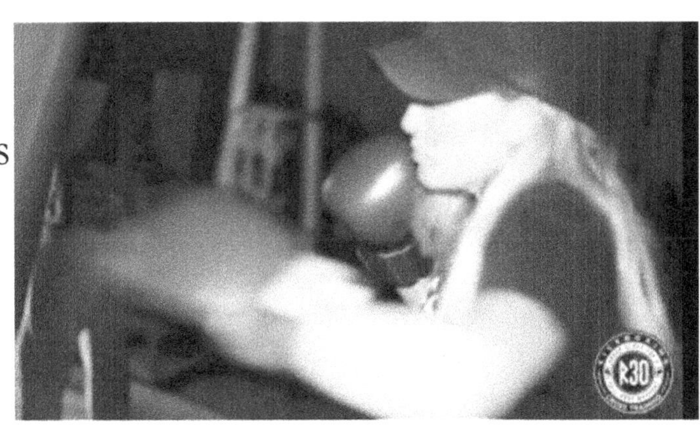

WORKOUT 18

Round 1 – Cardio
        50 Jump Rope
        20 High Knees

Round 2 – Weights (Legs)
        20 Alternating Reverse Lunges
        20 Sumo Squats

Round 3 – Heavy Bag Round
        1, 2, 3, 2, 2, 2, R Elbow
        Shuffle
        4 Instep Kicks

Round 4 -Weights (Chest & Tricep)
        15 Push Ups
        15 Tricep Pull Downs

Round 5 – Heavy Bag
        LRH, RRH, LRH 2,3,2
        Shuffle
        DOUBLE Jab

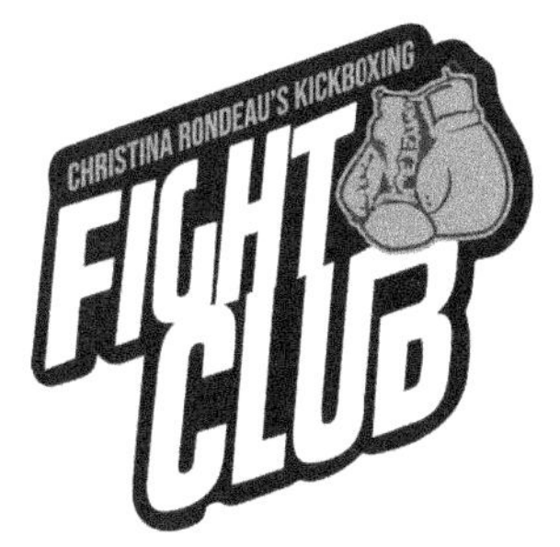

Round 6 - Speed Bag (Left Fighting Stance)
       10 L
       10 R
       20 Alternating

Round 7 – Heavy Bag Round
       1, 2, 3, 5 LRH, 2
       Shuffle
       10 Punches

Round 8 – Heavy Bag Round
       LRH, Right Axe Kick, Left RH 2,3,222
       Shuffle
       10 Alternating RH Kicks

Round 9 – Weights
       15 Ball Slams
       30 Toe Taps

Round 10 – Abs
       Full Sit UP W/
         2 punches at top
       10 Leg Lifts

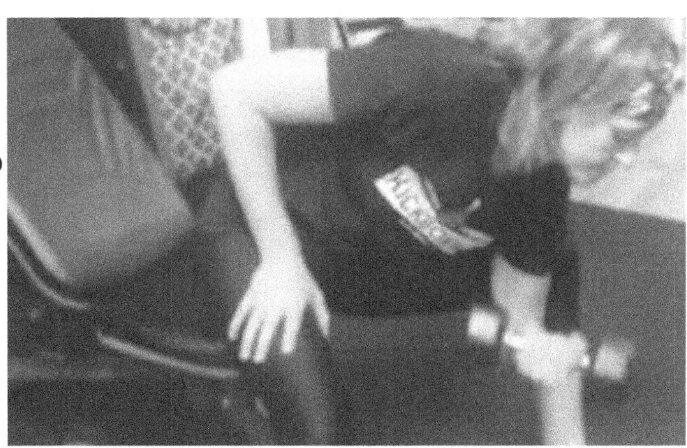

WORKOUT 19

Round 1 – Cardio
        10 Jump Squats
        25 Sumo Squats
        20 Alternating Curtsey Squats

Round 2 – Weights (Back & Shoulders)
        15 Bent Over Rows
        15 Reverse Fly's

Round 3 – Heavy Bag Round
        LRH, R-Instep, LRH 2,3,2
        Shuffle
        1, 2, 3, 4, 4, 4, 4 Alternating

Round 4 -Weights (Back & Bicep)
        10 TRX Rows
        10 Cable Rope Hammer Curls

Round 5 – Heavy Bag
        1, 2, 3, L-Back Fist 2
        Shuffle
        4 Instep Kicks

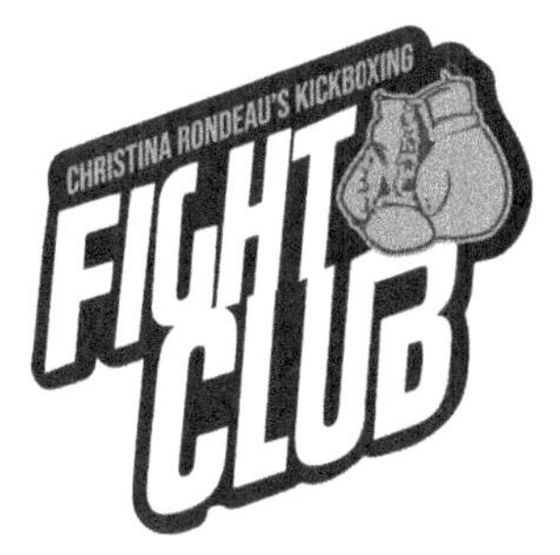

Round 6 - Speed Bag (Left Fighting Stance)
        20 L
        20 R
        20 Alternating

Round 7 – Heavy Bag Round
        1, 2, Reverse Backfist, 2,3,2
        Shuffle
        10 Straight Punches

Round 8 – Heavy Bag Round
        1, 5, LRH, 2, 2, 2, R Elbow
        Shuffle
        10 Alternating Kicks

Round 9 – Weights
        20 Mountain Climbers
        10 Inner Thigh Ball Squeeze
        10 Burpees

Round 10 – Abs
        25 Crunches
        25 Bicycles

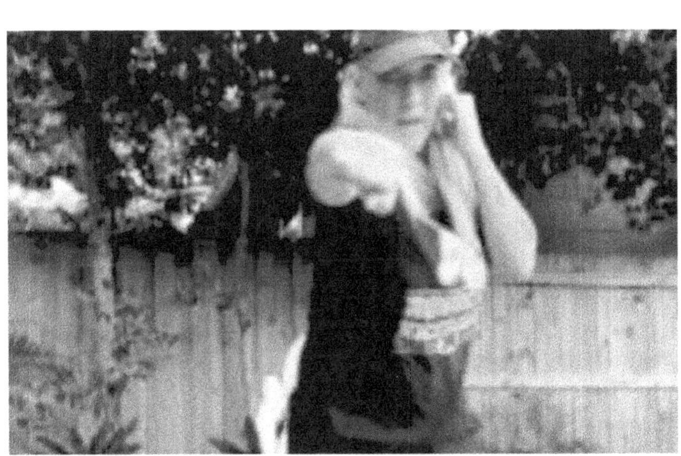

WORKOUT 20

Round 1 – Cardio
        Sprints Up and Down Room

Round 2 – Weights (Back and Biceps)
        15 Rows – Knee on Bench
        15 Circular Curls

Round 3 – Heavy Bag Round
        1, 1, L Backfist, 2, 3, 6, 3, 2
        Shuffle
        LRH, L Side Kick, LRH, 22

Round 4 -Weights (Shoulders & Biceps)
        12 Battle Ropes
        15 Straight Bar Curl

Round 5 – Heavy Bag
        1, 2, 1, 2, 3, 2
        Shuffle
        LRH, R Instep, LRH

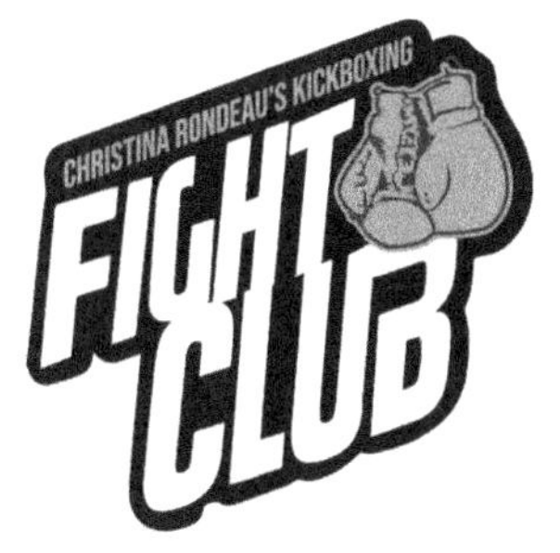

Round 6 - Speed Bag (Left Fighting Stance)
        20 L
        20 R
        20 Alternating

Round 7 – Heavy Bag Round
        1-2-3-5 LRH 2
        Shuffle
        10 Instep Kicks Alternating

Round 8 – Heavy Bag Round
        LRH, 5, 3, LRH, 2
        Shuffle
        1, 2, 3, 3, 6, 6

Round 9 – Weights (Chest)
        15 Chest Press
        15 Overhead Chest Extensions

Round 10 – Abs
        20 Crunches
        20 Flutter Kicks
        10 Leg Lifts

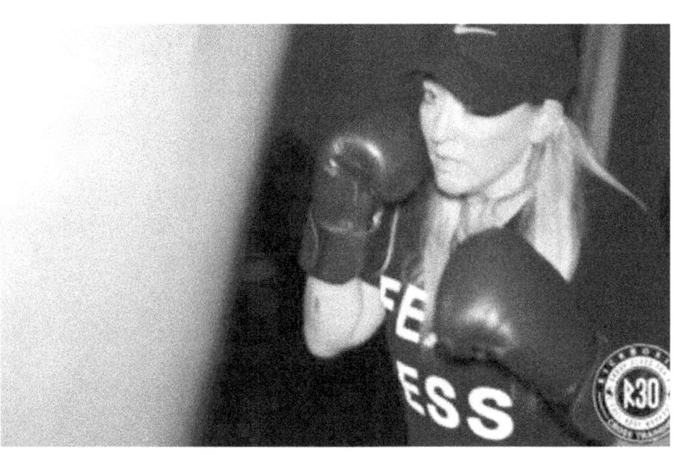

WORKOUT 21

Round 1 – Cardio
        30 Jump Rope
        10 Alternating Front Kicks

Round 2 – Weights (Chest & Triceps)
        12 Chest Press
        12 Tricep Kickbacks

Round 3 – Heavy Bag Round
        1, 2, 1, 2, 3, 2,
        Shuffle
        Body Hooks – 3 on each side

Round 4 -Weights (Triceps)
        12 Triceps Pull Downs
        12 Rope Overhead Extensions

Round 5 – Heavy Bag
        1, 2, 3, 6, 6, 3, 2
        Shuffle
        10 Alternating Round House Kicks

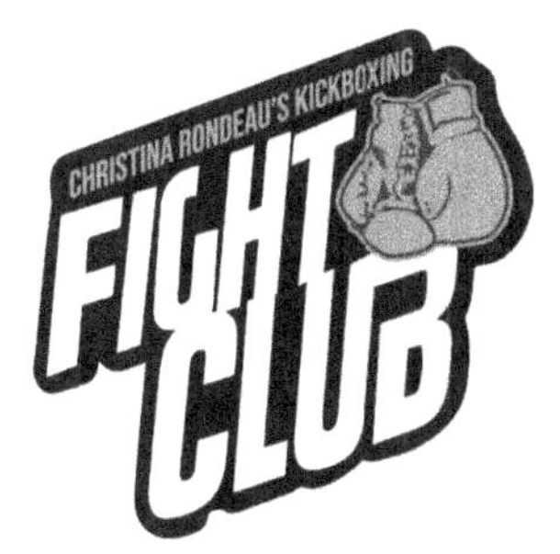

Round 6 - Speed Bag (Left Fighting Stance)
      20 R
      20 L
      20 Alternating

Round 7 – Heavy Bag Round
      10 Straight Punches
      10 Alternating Hooks
      10 Instep Kicks

Round 8 – Heavy Bag Round
      Jab, Double Back Fist, 2, 3, 2
      Shuffle
      2, 3, L Hammer, L Hammer, 2, 2, R Elbow

Round 9 – Weights
      12 Bosu Squat
      20 Courtesy Lunges

Round 10 – Abs
      20 Leg Lifts
      20 Ankle Taps
        (side to side)
      40 Crunches

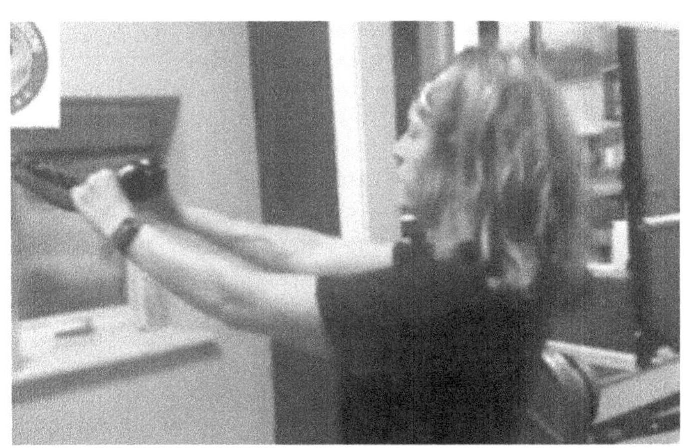

WORKOUT 22

Round 1 – Cardio
       20 Jumping Jacks
       20 Pushups

Round 2 – Weights (Shoulders)
       15 Front Lateral Raises
       15 Side Lateral Raises

Round 3 – Heavy Bag Round
       1, 2, 3, 4, 4, 4, 4
       Shuffle
       4 Instep Kicks

Round 4 -Weights (Back & Bicep)
       10 Upright Rows
       10 Bicep Curls

Round 5 – Heavy Bag
       1-3-1 2,4,2
       Shuffle
       10 Alternating RH Kicks

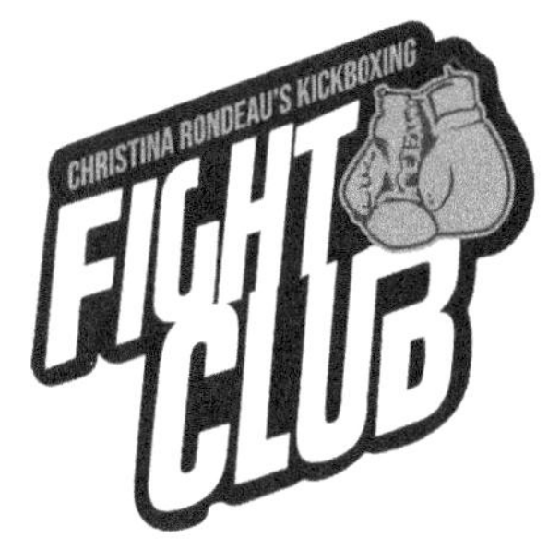

Round 6 - Speed Bag (Left Fighting Stance)
        3 L
        3 R

Round 7 – Heavy Bag Round
        1-2-3-2
        Shuffle
        LRH, LRH, R Instep Kick, RRH

Round 8 – Heavy Bag Round
        1, 2, 3, 5, LRH, 2
        Shuffle
        LRH, L-Side Kick, LRH

Round 9 – Weights
        10 Bosu Squats
        15 Bosu Bridges
        10 Bosu Plank Jacks

Round 10 – Abs
        10 Full Sit Ups
        20 Leg Lifts
        40 Bicycles

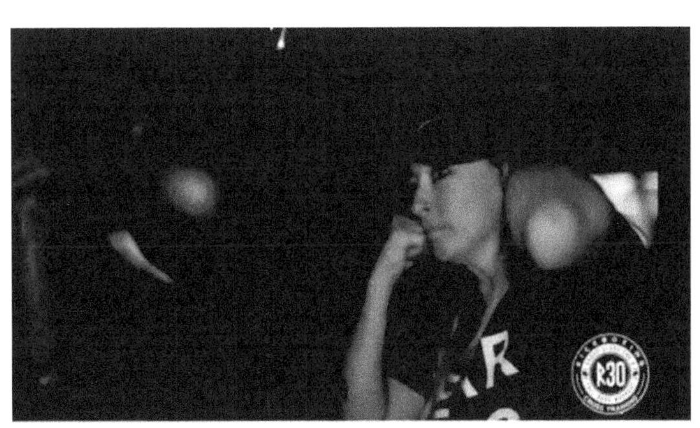

WORKOUT 23

Round 1 – Cardio
> 50 Toe Taps on Ball
> 20 Ball Slams

Round 2 – Weights (Chest & Tricep)
> 10 Incline Chest Flys
> 10 Seated Tricep Kickbacks

Round 3 – Heavy Bag Round
> 4 Ball Kicks
> Shuffle
> 1, 2, 3, 4, 3, 2

Round 4 -Weights (Chest & Tricep)
> 10 TRX Chest Press
> 10 Tricep Pull Downs

Round 5 – Heavy Bag
> L Backfist, R backfist, L backfirst, 2,3,2
> Shuffle
> 20 Punches

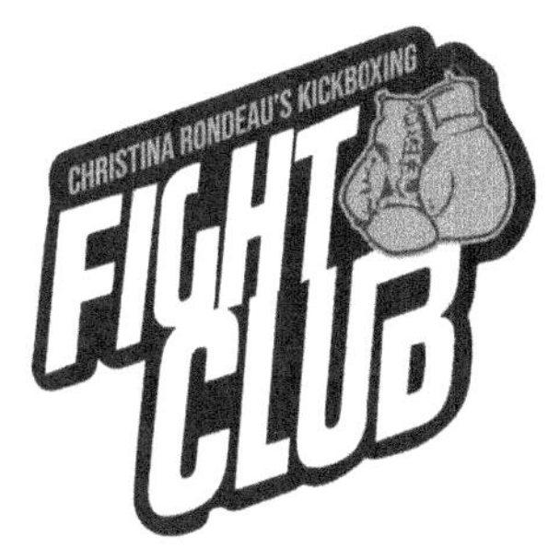

Round 6 - Speed Bag (Left Fighting Stance)
        3 Minutes – Mix it up

Round 7 – Heavy Bag
        10 Uppercuts
        Shuffle
        10 Hooks to Body

Round 8 – Heavy Bag Round
        1, 5, LRH, 2, 2, 2, Rt. Elbow
        Shuffle
        LRH, R Ball, L Ball, RRH

Round 9 – Weights
        15 Dead Lifts
        15 Ice Skaters

Round 10 – Abs
        25 Crunches
        25 Flutter Kicks

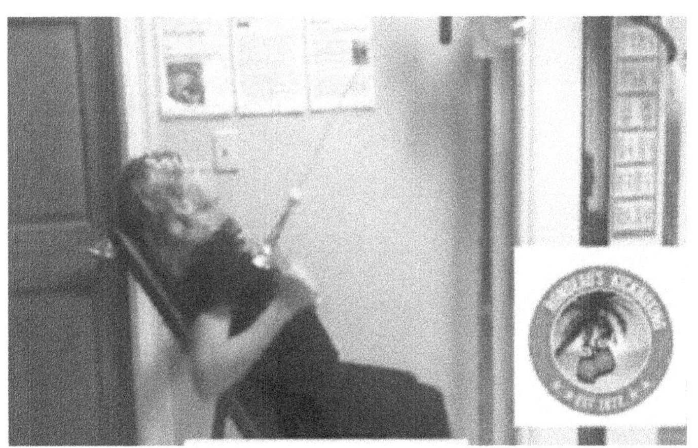

WORKOUT 24

Round 1 – Cardio
        20 Jump Squats
        20 Alt. Lunges

Round 2 – Weights (Back & Biceps)
        15 Seated Flys with Chest on Legs
        15 Hammer Curls

Round 3 – Heavy Bag Round
        20 Punches
        10 Instep Kicks

Round 4 -Weights (Shoulders and Biceps)
        12 Upright Row
        12 Straight Bar Curl

Round 5 – Heavy Bag
        Double Jab
        Shuffle
        1, 2, 3, 6, 3, 2

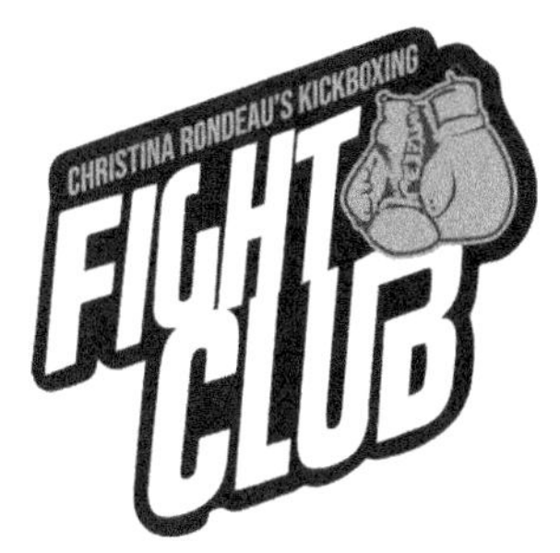

Round 6 - Speed Bag (Left Fighting Stance)
        10 Left
        10 Right
        20 Alternating

Round 7 – Heavy Bag Round
        1-3-1 2-6-2
        Shuffle
        LRH, L Instep Kick, R Instep Kick, RRH

Round 8 – Heavy Bag Round
        10 Alternating Hooks
        10 Alternating Round House Kicks

Round 9 – Weights
        15 Kettle Bell RDL
        15 Kettle Bell One Arm Military Press

Round 10 – Abs
        20 Crunches
        20 Bicycles
        20 Leg Lifts

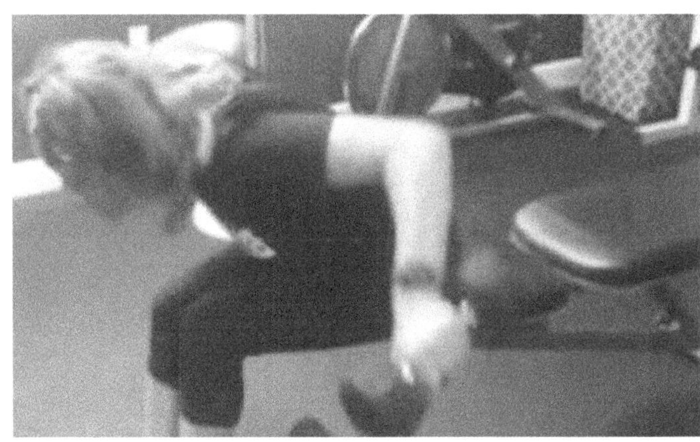

WORKOUT 25

Round 1 – Cardio
Shadow Box w/ weights

Round 2 – Weights (Back & Bicep)
12 Bicep Curls
12 Upright Rows

Round 3 – Heavy Bag Round
1, 3, 1, 2, 6, 2
Shuffle
10 Alternating Instep Kicks

Round 4 -Weights (Back & Bicep)
12 Lat Pulldowns
12 Single Bicep Curls each arm

Round 5 – Heavy Bag
1, 2, 3, 2, 2, RRH, R Elbow
Shuffle
LRH, R Instep, LRH

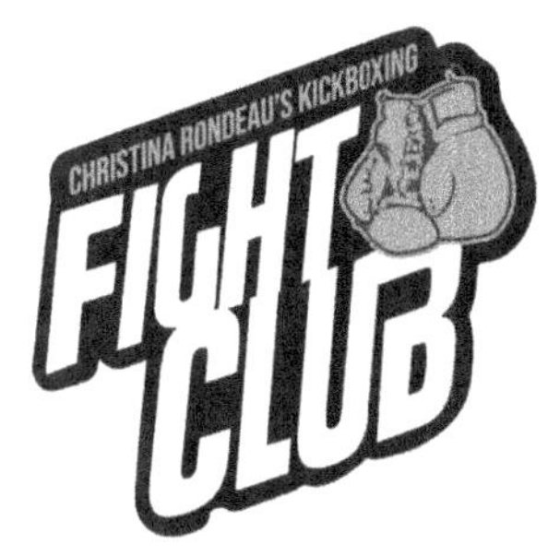

Round 6 - Speed Bag (Left Fighting Stance)
   3 L
   3 R

Round 7 – Heavy Bag Round
   1, 2, 3, 6, 3, 2,
   Shuffle
   20 Punches

Round 8 – Heavy Bag Round
   1, 2, 3, 5, LRH, 2
   Shuffle
   RRH, RRH

Round 9 – Weights
   15 Squat Curl Press
   15 Lunges with a bicep curl

Round 10 – Abs
   10 Sit ups
   20 Leg Lifts
   30 Bicycles

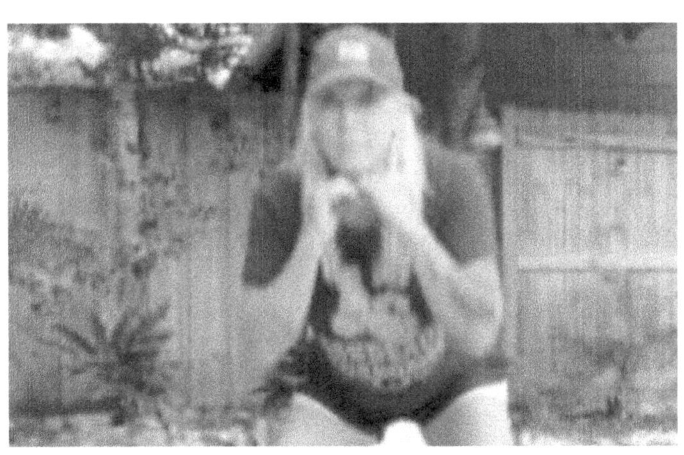

WORKOUT 26

Round 1 – Cardio
      Agility Ladder
      In and Outs

Round 2 – Weights (Full Body)
      10 Squat W/ Bicep Curl on Top
      12 Front Shoulder Raises

Round 3 – Heavy Bag Round
      6 Instep Kicks
      Shuffle
      LRH, RRH, LRH, 2,3, 2

Round 4 -Weights (Chest and Triceps)
      15 Cable Cross Over
      15 One Arm Cable Press Down

Round 5 – Heavy Bag
      1, 2, 3, 4, 3, 2
      Shuffle
      RRH, RRH, LRH, LRH, 2

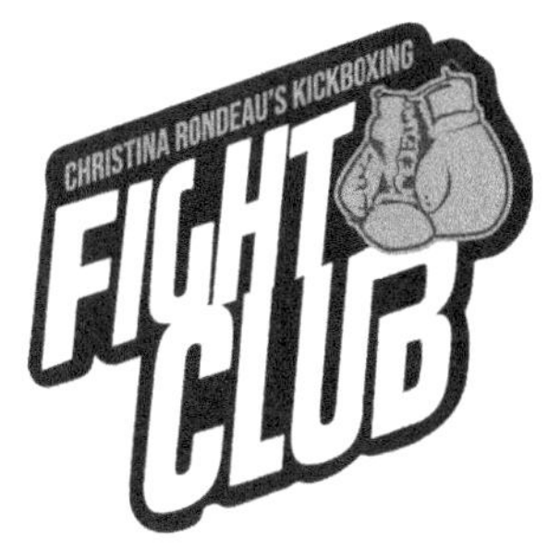

Round 6 - Speed Bag (Left Fighting Stance)
      20 L
      20 R
      20 Alternating

Round 7 – Heavy Bag Round
      1, 2, 3, 2, 3, 2
      Shuffle
      10 Punches

Round 8 – Heavy Bag Round
      1, 3, 1, 2, 6, 2
      Shuffle
      LRH, RRH, LRH, 2, 2, 2, RH Elbow

Round 9 – Weights
      10 Burpees
      10 Push Ups

Round 10 – Abs
      20 Mountain
        Climbers
      20 Bicycles

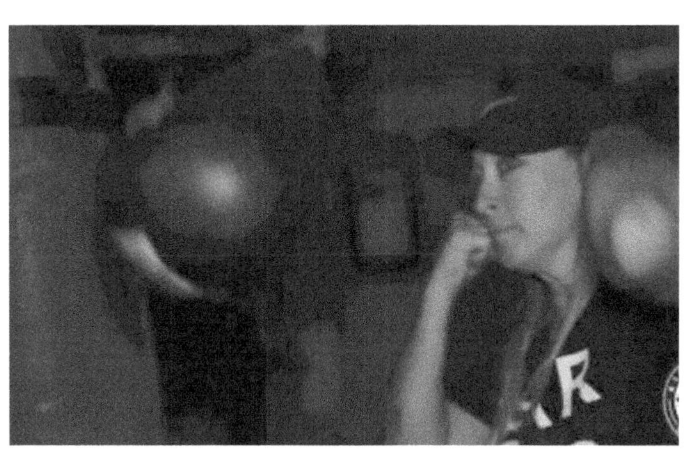

WORKOUT 27

Round 1 – Cardio
       20 Corner to Corner Knee Ups on Step
       20 Jump Ups on Box
       20 Push Ups

Round 2 – Weights (Shoulders)
       15 Around the World w/ Front Raises
       15 Shoulder Presses

Round 3 – Heavy Bag Round
       10 Straight Punches 1, 2
       Shuffle
       LRH, RRH, LRH, 2

Round 4 -Weights (Back & Bicep)
       15 Lateral Pull Down
       15 Straight Bar Bicep Curls

Round 5 – Heavy Bag
       1, 2, 3, 5, LRH, 2, 3, 2
       Shuffle
       4 Punches

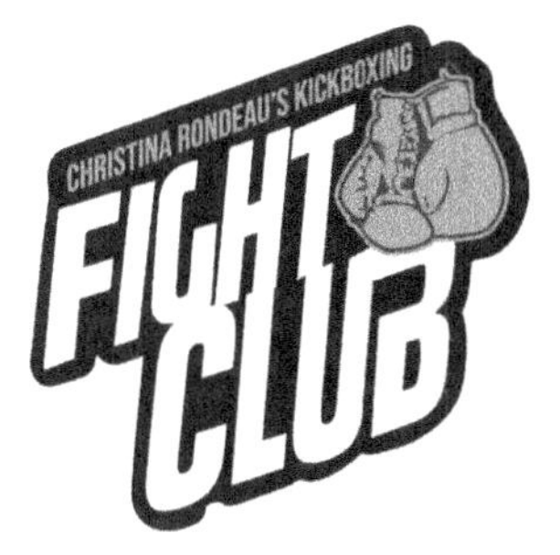

Round 6 - Speed Bag (Left Fighting Stance)
      20 L
      20 R
      20 Alternating

Round 7 – Heavy Bag Round
      1, 2, 3, 2, 3, 2,
      Shuffle
      RRH, RRH, LRH, LRH

Round 8 – Heavy Bag Round
      LRH, R Front Ball Kick , LRH
      Shuffle
      1, 3, 1, 2, 4, 2, R-Elbow

Round 9 – Weights
      Squats with Ball, Toss on Top
      20 Palm Strikes

Round 10 – Abs
      20 Leg Lifts
      Crunches w/ Ball

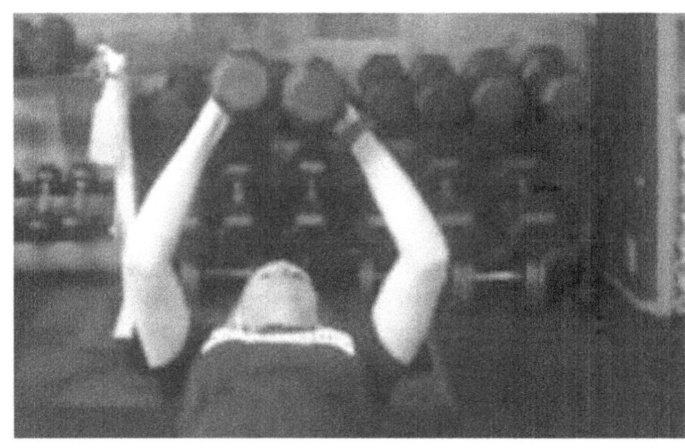

WORKOUT 28

Round 1 – Cardio
  20 Squats
  20 Jumping Jacks
  20 Air Jump Rope

Round 2 – Weights (Chest)
  12 Chest Press
  12 Overhead Raise

Round 3 – Heavy Bag Round
  1, 2, 1, 2
  Shuffle
  4 Front Ball Kicks

Round 4 -Weights (Legs)
  12 TRX Squats
  Rope Cable Pull Throughs

Round 5 – Heavy Bag
  1-2- Reverse Backfist 2-3-2
  Shuffle
  10 Punches

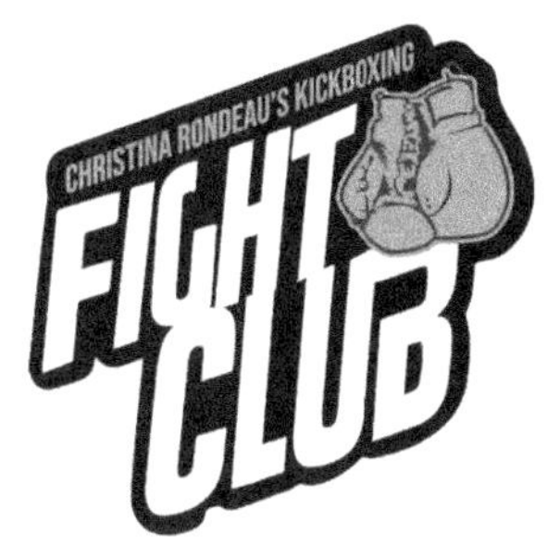

Round 6 - Speed Bag
        10 L
        10 R

Round 7 – Heavy Bag Round
        1 Slip 2, 3, 2
        Shuffle
        20 Punches

Round 8 – Heavy Bag Round
        1, 5, Left Roundhouse 2, 3, 2
        Shuffle
        Double Jab

Round 9 – Weights
        15 Squat Curl Press
        15 Hammer Curls

Round 10 – Abs
        30 Mountain Climbers
        30 Bicycles

WORKOUT 29

Round 1 – Cardio
      10 Back Side Step W/ Kick
      15 Jump Squats
      20 Instep Kicks

Round 2 – Weights (Bicep & Shoulder)
      12 Military Press
      12 Bicep Curls

Round 3 – Heavy Bag Round
      1, 2, 3, 1
      8 Instep Kicks

Round 4 -Weights (Back)
      12 Lat Pull Downs
      12 Face Pulls

Round 5 – Heavy Bag
      1, 3, 1, 2, 4, 2
      Shuffle
      LRH, RRH, LRH, RRH

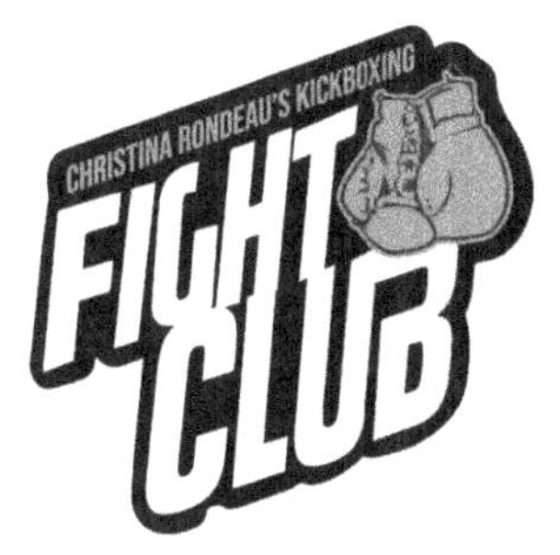

Round 6 - Speed Bag (Left Fighting Stance)
        5 L - 5R
        3 L - 3R
        1 L - 1R

Round 7 – Heavy Bag Round
        1-2-U -2 -3-2
        Shuffle
        6 Alternating Instep Kicks

Round 8 – Heavy Bag Round
        10 Cross Behind Side Kicks Right Leg
        10 Cross Behind Side Kicks Left Leg

Round 9 – Weights
        15 Ball Slams
        30 Toe Taps

Round 10 – Abs
        20 Crunches
        20 Flutter Kicks
        Hold Low Leg
           Lift for least
           30 sec.

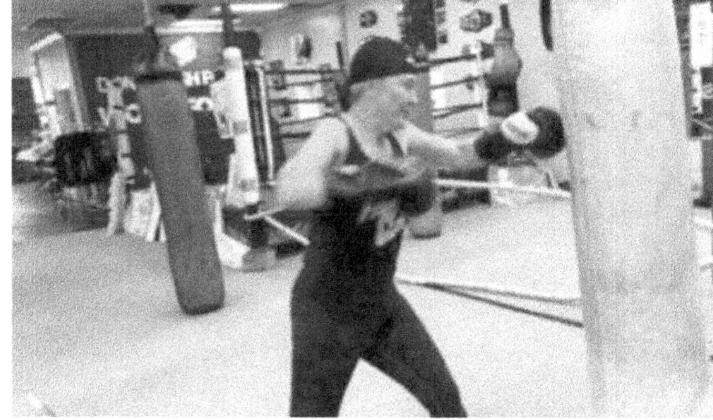

WORKOUT 30

Round 1 – Cardio
        2 Minutes Jump Rope
        1 Minute Straight Punches W/ Weights

Round 2 – Weights (Back & Bicep)
        12 Back Fly's
        12 Hammer Curls

Round 3 – Heavy Bag Round
        1, 2, 3, 2, LRH, 2
        Shuffle
        6 Instep Kicks, 2

Round 4 -Weights (Back & Bicep)
        15 Lateral Pull down
        15 Bicep Curls with Rope

Round 5 – Heavy Bag
        1, 3, 1, 2, 4, 2, 2,
        Shuffle
        LRH, RRH, LRH

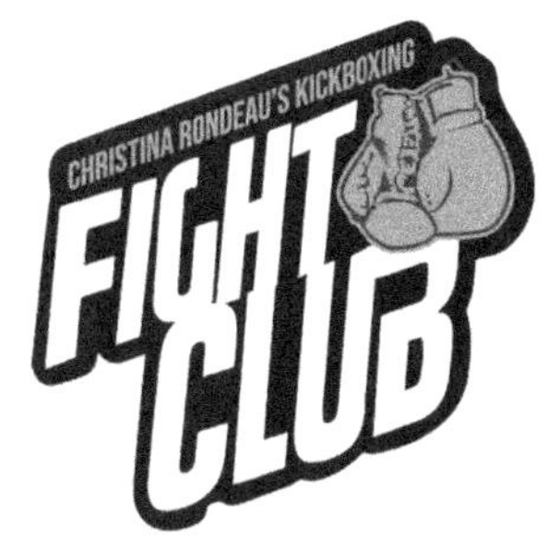

Round 6 - Speed Bag (Left Fighting Stance)
        L 20
        R 20
        Alternating 20

Round 7 – Heavy Bag Round
        1, 2, 3, 5, 3, 2
        Shuffle
        20 Straight Punches

Round 8 – Heavy Bag Round
        1 double backfist 2, 3, 2
        Shuffle
        10 Punches

Round 9 – Weights
        10 Squat Jacks
        20 Toe Taps on Ball
        10 Kettle Bell Swings

Round 10 – Abs
        20 Plank w/
            Shoulder Taps
        20 Full Situps
        20 Crunches

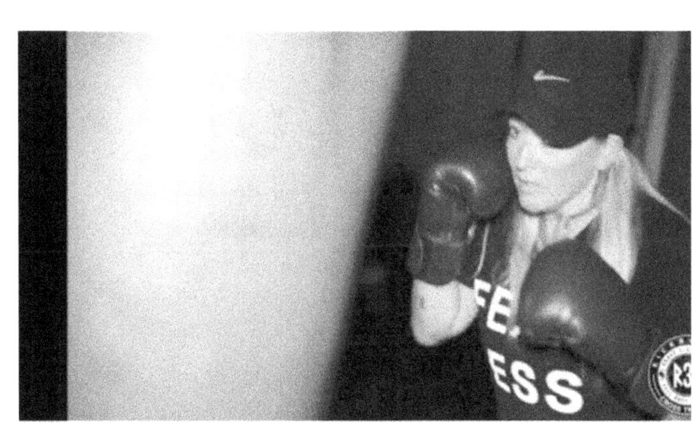

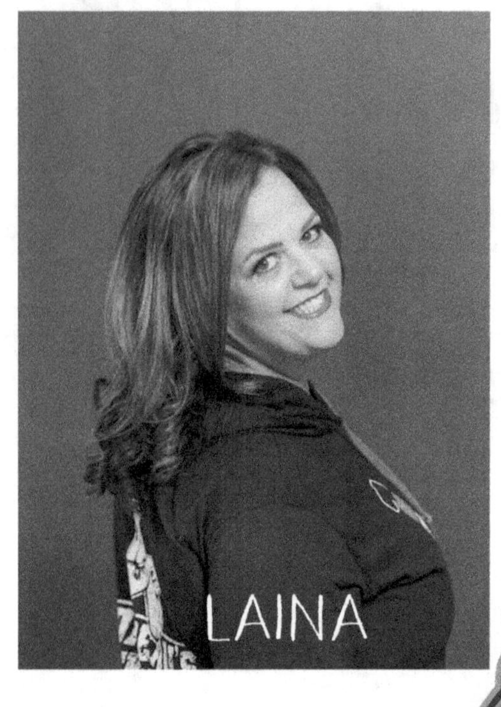

LAINA

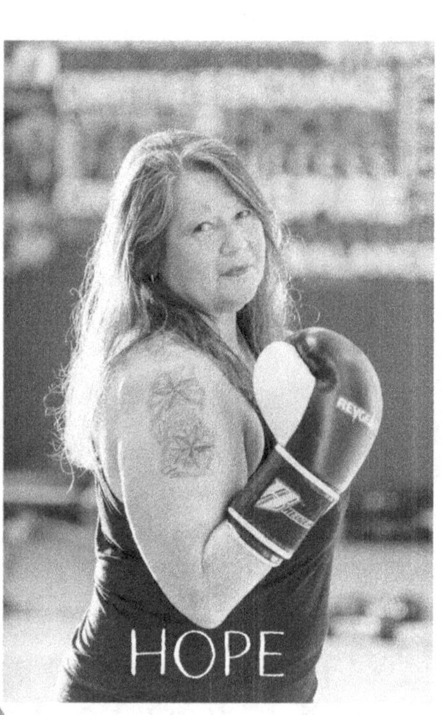

HOPE

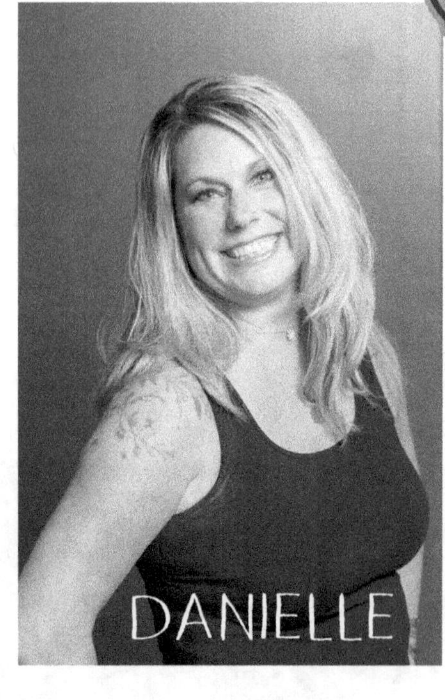

DANIELLE

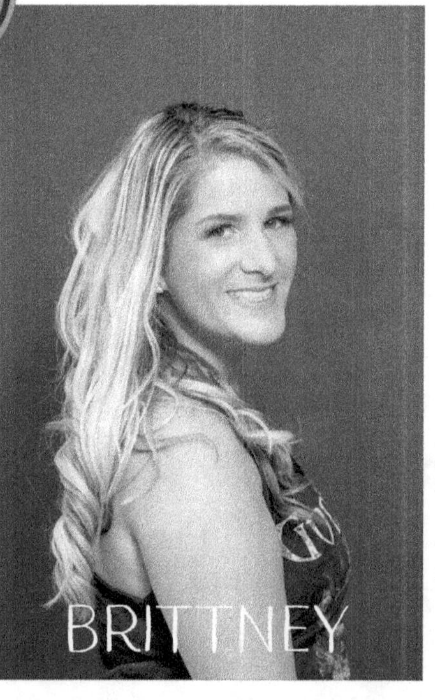

BRITTNEY

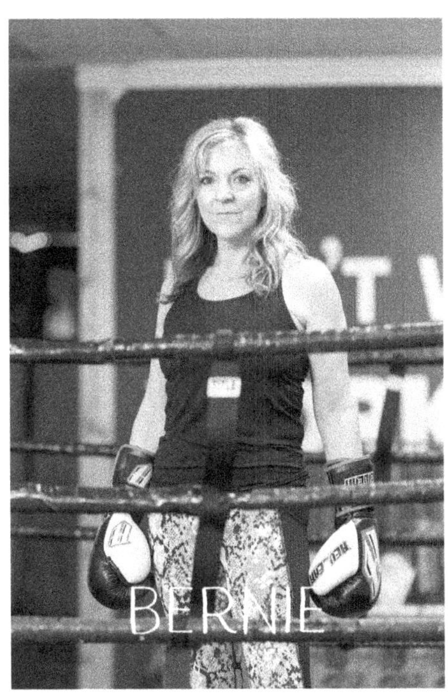
BERNIE

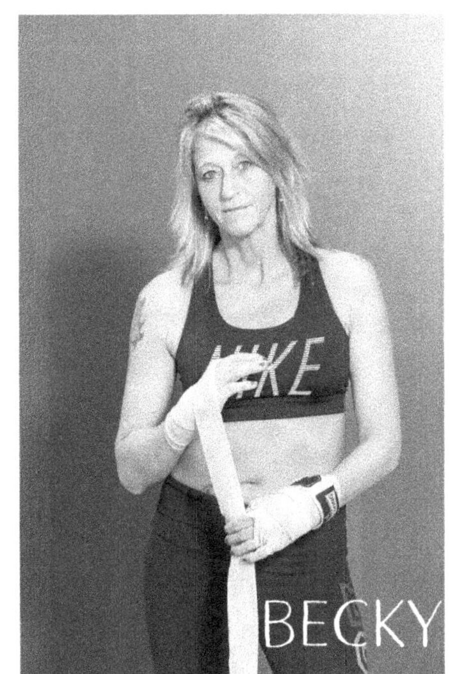
BECKY

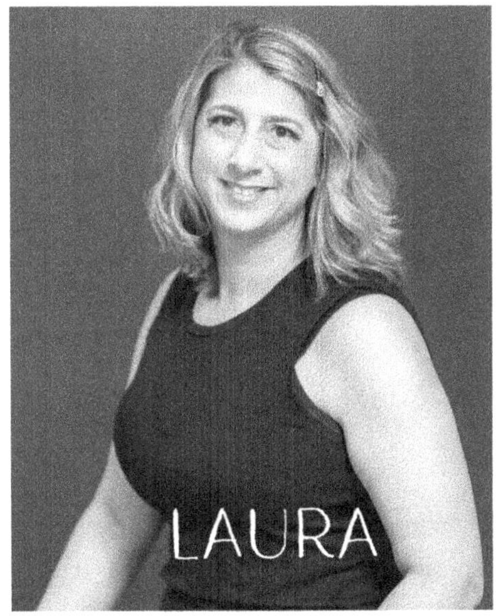
LAURA

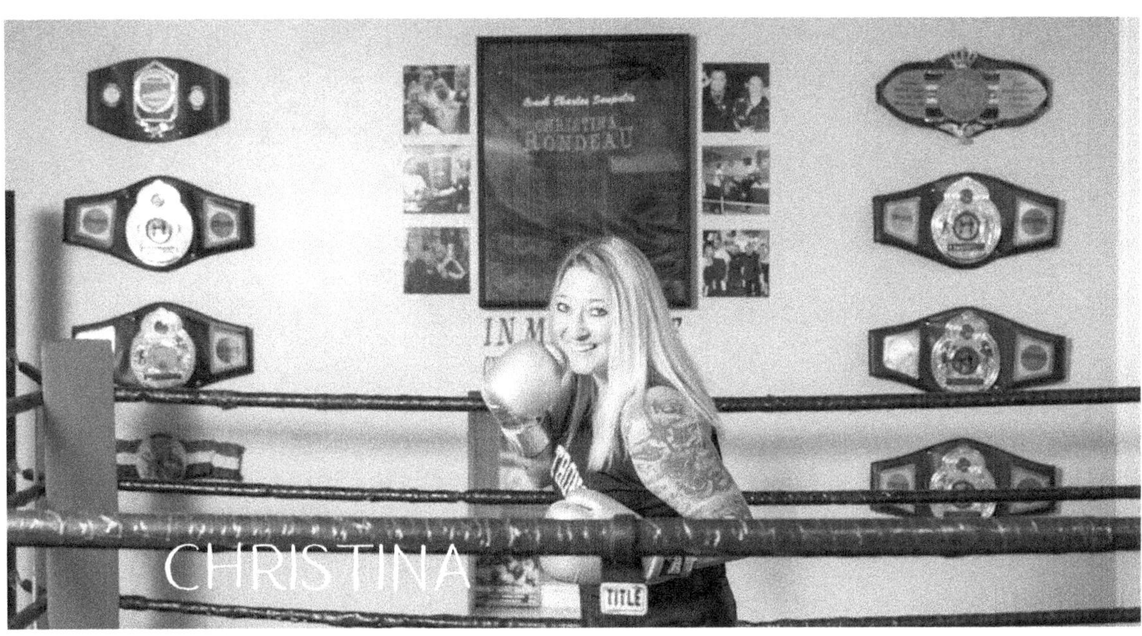
CHRISTINA

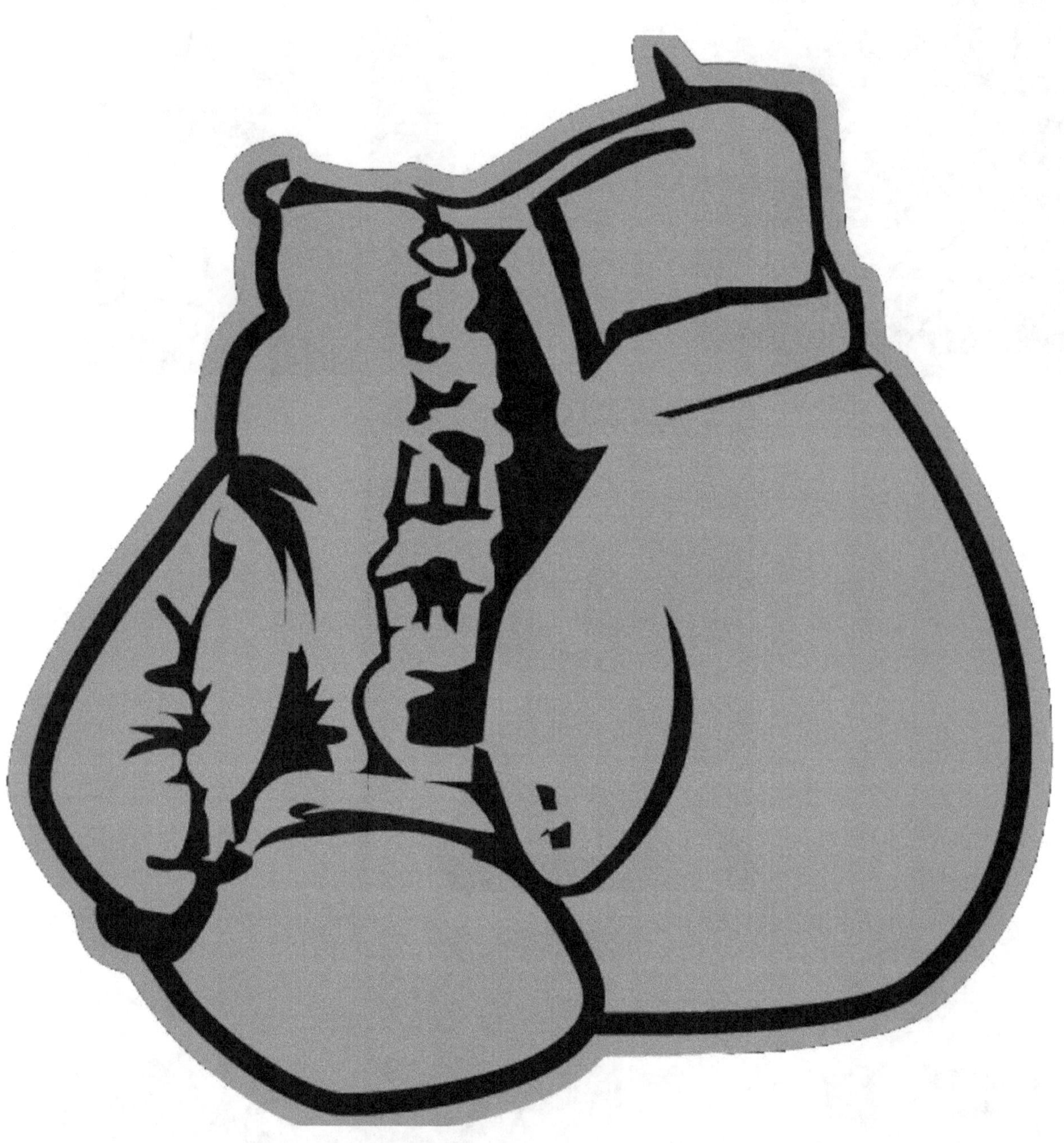